# STEP TRAINING PLUS
# THE WAY TO FITNESS
## SECOND EDITION

**Lauren M. Mangili, M.Ed.**
University of North Carolina, Chapel Hill

**Karen S. Mazzeo, M.Ed.**
Bowling Green State University

**Morton Publishing Company**
925 West Kenyon Avenue, Unit 12
Englewood, Colorado 80110
http://www.morton-pub-com

Typography by Ash Street Typecrafters, Inc., Denver, Colorado
Cover Design by Bob Schram, Bookends, Inc., Boulder, Colorado
Illustrations by Susan Strawn, Loveland, Colorado
Edited by Carolyn Acheson, Aurora, Colorado
Cover Photo Photography by Erik Perel, Chapel Hill, North Carolina
Interior Photography by Jeffrey Hall Photography, Haskins, Ohio and
Erik Perel, Chapel Hill, North Carolina.

Copyright © 1999, Morton Publishing Company
ISBN: 0-89582-458-2

10 9 8 7 6 5 4 3 2 1

Printed in the United States of America

# ACKNOWLEDGMENTS

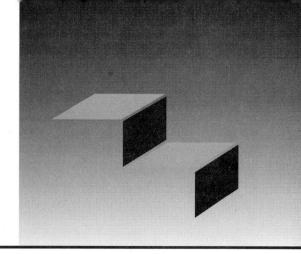

*Special appreciation to the following individuals who have shared their time and superior talents in this endeavor:*

Jamy Albo
Todd Belknap
Dr. Kathy Browder
"Colton" at Gateway
Linda Contreras
Sharon Denny
Stephen Gagnon
Philip H. Goldstein
Jeffery L. Hall
Nancy Hamsik
Peter Holmes
Ruth Horton
Virnette D. House
Vanya C. Jones
Alisson Kallenbach
Tammy Kime-Sheets, R.D.

Pam Kosanke
Mary Beth Mazzeo
Dr. Robert McMurray
Douglas N. Morton
Saudia Muhammed
Peggy Paul, R.D., L.D.
Erik Perel
Dr. William E. Prentice
Dr. Bernard Rabin
Laura Reiger
Joanne R. Saliger
Carrie Robinson Sanderson
Vivian Smallwood
Mary Teachey
David Thornton
John Virostek

*Appreciation to the following for granting permission to use copyrighted materials:*

The American Dietetics Association and *The Journal of the American Dietetics Association*

Kenneth Cooper, M.D., M.P.H., and Bantam/Doubleday/Dell

Oregon Dairy Council

Werner W. K. Hoeger, Ph.D., and Morton Publishing Company

YMCA of the USA

William Prentice, and McGraw Hill Publishing Company

*A special thank you to the following companies for providing apparel and equipment with which to photograph:*

Nike, Inc., One Bowerman Drive, Beaverton, OR 97005
(1-800-535-6453) for fitness apparel

Every day is a gift, and every day I give thanks. I am thankful for all the gifts I have been given — a loving, supportive family and caring friends who help make my dreams possible.

*Lauren*

To my cadre of earthbound angels, BeverlyK* CarolynP* CharlesT* CraigM* DanZ* DickM* DorothyP* DougM* EdW* EugeniaA* JessicaO* JimR* KarenT* LindaC* MargoC* MariaC* MarilynB* MaryBethM* MelvaL* MichaelM* MojaK* PatJ* RobertaK* ShirleyMc* SueS* TammyKS*. You have inspired my spirit and abundantly and unconditionally provided your talents and gifts just when I've needed them! Your loving, giving natures feed my soul. Thank you.

*Karen*

# CONTENTS

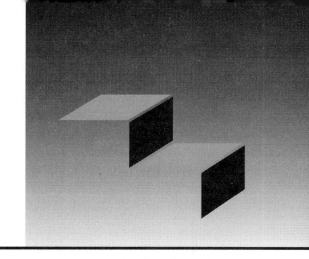

# INTRODUCTION

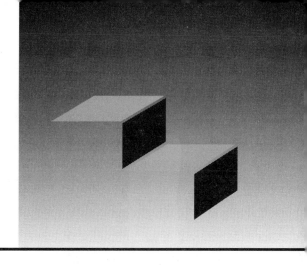

Bench/step training, or step training, is continuing its immense popularity with fitness professionals and enthusiasts into the 21st century. Step training, which uses a 4" to 12" step bench, is a safe and efficient method for achieving and maintaining physical fitness. Many participants consider it their top choice of modality for working out, and *the* way to fitness for a lifetime!

*Step Training Plus: The Way to Fitness,* Second Edition, updates the latest fitness research available. It assists individuals like yourself, who are taking physical fitness courses, to understand the basic principles and techniques involved in step training. The "Plus" tells how to structure a total physical fitness and mental training workout that will motivate you to make healthy choices for a lifetime.

*Step Training Plus* is designed for the novice requiring the basics and for the instructor-to-be to understand the methods behind the basics. Its brief, easy-to-follow, sequential learning order can be the map and compass for one's journey toward personal fitness excellence.

The three-hole punched book format allows for greater ease and flexibility of use by the student enrolled in a fitness course, as well as the instructor who may choose to provide additional handout pages of researched information and techniques to be taught. Students are encouraged to use this text as a personalized workbook, continually assessing their starting points, monitoring their progress and change, and setting goals to work toward. Pages can easily be removed and submitted to the instructor for review and evaluation, and then returned to their original locations within the text for continual reference during the course and for years to come.

This second edition is divided into two sections, I and II. Section I begins with two forms entitled, *Student Information Profile* and *Student Physical Activity Readiness.* The information

gathered serves as part of the prescreening for both fitness testing and exercise participation. Section I continues by addressing all of the principles, techniques, and options for the exciting step training program in Chapters 1 through 8.

Chapter 1 initiates *A Step In The Right Direction* by presenting total fitness principles and definitions. These lay a broad foundation for understanding the specific fitness techniques you will be using.

Chapter 2 encourages you to take *The First Step.* Using the information obtained in the prescreening forms, this chapter helps you describe your starting point — where you are today — through testing procedures that are easily conducted in a class setting. From there, you'll be able to establish program goals, monitor your progress, and see your results.

Chapter 3 invites you to take *The Next Step* in understanding the specific fitness activity called step training. It covers the benefits, latest research, how to choose your bench height and music tempo, proper alignment and technique, positions to avoid, shoe selection, and general safety precautions.

Chapter 4 presents the *Segments of a Step Class* and specific information to consider while participating in each. The four segments are: warm-up, step aerobics, strength/muscle conditioning, and the cool-down, flexibility, and relaxation segment. The types of movements, music tempo, and length of each segment are recommended.

Chapter 5 takes you *Step By Step* through the basic techniques of step training. The techniques are described with photographs using the "mirrored" method for all *front* views. A movement described and visualized as using the left foot/arm/or side of the body shown is actually the right foot/arm/side of the model (see Figure I.1). Therefore, you do not have to reverse the direction of what is pictured and described and what you are to perform. You simply perform the

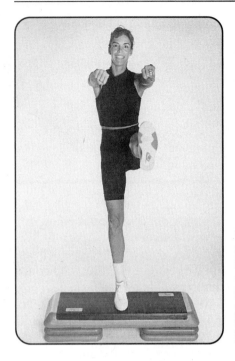

**Figure I.1.** Stepping up onto the bench, taking weight on your **left** foot, kick your **right** leg forward, waist-high.

movement on the same side of the body as you see it photographed and described. (Movement photographed from the model's *side* view or *rear* view are natural and not "mirrored"; right and left steps are the same as the model's right and left.)

Creativity is fostered in Chapter 6 by giving you a chance to *Step to the Beat* — providing you the framework for putting moves together. Principles of balance, selecting and sequencing movements, transitions, and adding variety are presented. This chapter offers ideas on how to safely progress through a step program (beginner to advanced stepper and simple to complex movements). By varying the intensity, you are sufficiently and continually challenged according to your own fitness level, skill level, current health status, and goals you've set. The advanced options in this chapter can provide a goal for the beginner to aspire to, and that occasional needed change for continually challenging the trained stepper. Ways to build unlimited possibilities are also provided, along with a worksheet to apply what you've learned.

Chapter 7 presents *A Step Ahead,* adding variety to your program once you've learned the basics.

It includes format options, methods for combination training using other fitness modalities such as slide, jump rope and sports conditioning, and efficient training techniques you can use to enhance your step training program. Having progressed to being an intermediate-to-advanced stepper, variety in the workout format becomes a *plus* to stay motivated and to continue to adhere to this or any other training modality.

Chapter 8 features *A Stronger Step,* emphasizing strength and endurance training of the skeletal muscles using the bench in level, incline, and decline positions, in conjunction with a variety of resistance equipment.

Section II details the *Plus* in the title, including numerous additional areas of awareness, education, assessment, and monitoring one needs to consider when taking a course that emphasizes the development of a *total* fitness lifestyle. This section emphasizes making the mind-body-spirit connection necessary for one's total well-being.

If you personally have difficulty starting a physical fitness program, you may want to begin the course in Section II, reading Chapter 9 first. This chapter will provide the principles and techniques needed immediately for understanding how internal *Motivation and Goal Setting* can work successfully for you now. For participants eager to get right into the physical step training principles and techniques, this mental training chapter will likely be presented later in your course, to solidify lifetime compliance to your program.

*Nutrition* is one of the hottest interest topics today and, therefore, is greatly expanded in Chapter 10. Variety and quantity of foods to eat and drink, nutrient density, vegetarian eating, and thirst replenishment are only a few of the many concepts presented.

Chapter 11 takes a look at the *Weight Management* issues of fat loss, lean gain, and weight maintenance. It explains assessment of body composition and offers several positive ideas to consider if changes are needed.

The steps toward lifetime fitness are taken one at a time beginning now, in the present moment. All steps become easier, quicker, and automatic if they are considered *fun.* Enjoy your fitness journey!

# SECTION 1

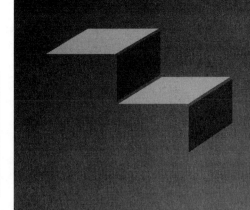

**LEVEL 4**    Limit...
- sitting
- watching TV

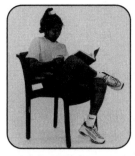

**LEVEL 3**

2–3 days/week

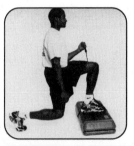

Flexibility

Muscular strength/
endurance

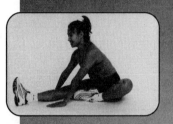

**LEVEL 2**

3–5 days/week moderate intensity

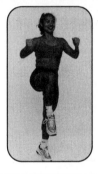

Aerobic
activities
- aerobic dance
- jogging
- biking

Recreational
activities
- racquetball
- basketball
- tennis

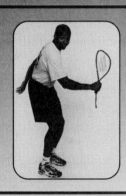

**LEVEL 1**    Choose to be active every day!
- use the stairs ▪ park further from destination ▪ walk the dog

---

The four levels of the fitness pyramid may be used as a guide for developing a well balanced fitness program. The bottom layer of the pyramid encourages you to be active by doing things for yourself rather than relying on modern conveniences. For example, when given a choice between taking the elevator or using the stairs, or walking instead of driving, choose to be active.

The second layer from the bottom promotes aerobic activities (aerobic dance, jogging, biking, step training) and recreational activities (basketball, tennis, racquetball, as examples) to strengthen the cardiovascular system.

The third level of the pyramid includes a flexibility and strength component, as well as leisure activities such as golf, bowling and yard work (that often are not as strenuous as aerobic exercise and vigorous recreational activities). These should be done a minimum of 2 or 3 days a week.

Finally, when constructing your fitness program, the top of the pyramid indicates an individual who lives a fit lifestyle and limits the amount of sitting and watching TV.

## ACSM Guidelines:

To achieve *cardiovascular benefits,* the American College of Sports Medicine (ACSM) recommends exercising 3 to 5 days a week at moderate to vigorous intensity, for 20 minutes or more. To improve *muscular strength and endurance,* ACSM recommends strength training 2 days per week, performing eight to ten exercises at approximately 70% to 85% of your one-repetition maximum.

# Personal Fitness Program

Name:_____Date:_____

1. Do you currently exercise? _____ No      _____ Yes

   If yes, how many days per week? _____

2. If yes, what type of exercises are you performing? _____

3. If you are not currently exercising, how long has it been since you have exercised? _____

   _____

4. List in numerical order the top three to five reasons you wish to become involved in a regular exercise program:

   _____Improve cardiovascular fitness      _____Reduce stress

   _____Lose fat weight      _____Gain lean weight

   _____Increase flexibility      _____Sleep better

   _____Improve muscular endurance      _____Increase energy

   _____Improve posture and appearance      _____Specific sport training:

   _____Increase muscular strength      List sport _____

5. Check the aerobic exercise machines you are familiar with:

   _____Climbmax      _____Cybex Bike      _____Nordic Track

   _____Concept II Rower      _____Freeclimber      _____Treadmill

   _____Crossrobics      _____Lifecycle

6. Check the weight machines you are familiar with:

   _____Cybex      _____Free Weights      _____Hammer

7. Check the aerobic exercises you enjoy:

   _____Aerobic dance      _____Jogging      _____Stair Stepping      _____Walking

   _____Cross-country Skiing      _____Jump Rope      _____Step Training

   _____Cycling      _____Rowing      _____Swimming Laps

8. What days of the week do you prefer to exercise?

   _____M      _____T      _____W      _____Th      _____F      _____Sat      _____Sun

9. What time of day do you plan to exercise?

   _____Early morning (6 a.m.–9 a.m.)      _____Evening (6 p.m.–9 p.m.)

   _____Mid morning (9 a.m.–noon)      _____Late night (9 p.m.–midnight)

   _____Early afternoon (noon–3 p.m.)

   _____Late afternoon (3 p.m.–6 p.m.)

10. How do you prefer to exercise?

    _____Alone      _____With a partner      _____In a group setting.

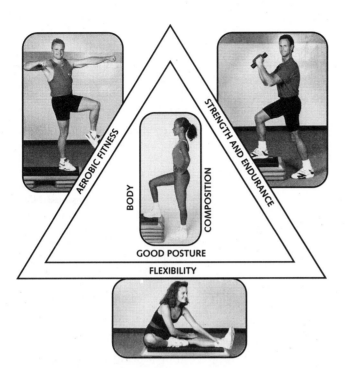

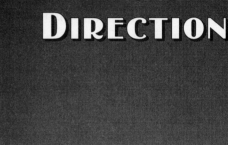
**B**y engaging in a physical fitness activity such as *aerobic* step training, you've taken the first step of your journey toward a meaningful, active lifestyle. Physical conditioning through step aerobics offers you a happier, more vivacious and abundant life. The physically fit active lifestyle actually prolongs life.[1] Furthermore,

> some predictions are that by the end of this century, the average American woman will live to age ninety, and the average American man to the mid-eighties.[2]

With these impressive findings and a projected long life ahead of us, let's make sure it will be a *quality* long life we're living (not just doing time), by making good choices.

Most simply stated, the term *aerobic means promoting the supply and use of oxygen.* The body's demand for oxygen increases when you engage in vigorous activity that produces specific beneficial changes in the body. *Aerobic, therefore, can refer to any type of exercise mode as long as it meets certain basic criteria.*

*Step training or step aerobics is an exercise mode that fulfills all of the criteria for aerobic exercise established by the American College of Sports Medicine.*

### A Total Physical Fitness Conditioning Program

Total physical fitness is the positive state of well-being allowing you enough strength and energy to participate in a full, active lifestyle of your choice. According to the American Medical Association, it is

> the general capacity to adapt favorably to physical effort. Individuals are physically fit when they are able to meet both the usual and unusual demands of daily life, safely and effectively without undue stress or exhaustion.

A total physical fitness conditioning program consists of five basic components. This can be visualized by the fitness triangle, depicting the three action components, plus the two structural components.

1. *Aerobic fitness* (cardiovascular and respiratory)
2. *Flexibility* (ability to bend and stretch)
3. *Muscular strength and muscular endurance* (thickening muscle fiber mass to enable individuals to endure a heavier workload)
4. *Good posture* (holding body in proper position for safety and efficiency)
5. *Body composition* (maintaining the proper fat weight-to-lean weight ratio).

A total, well-rounded weekly fitness conditioning program should consist of regular participation in all five components.

## Aerobic Fitness

Because the sign of genuine fitness is the condition of the heart, blood vessels, and lungs, aerobic fitness is the most important component. *Aerobic* exercise is exercise that requires oxygen for extended periods and demands an uninterrupted work output from your muscles. Aerobic exercise trains the heart, lungs, and cardiovascular system to deliver oxygen quickly and efficiently to every part of the body. The higher your fitness level, the better able your cardiovascular system is to deliver adequate oxygen. Endurance activities that are rhythmic, dynamic, continuous, and use large muscle groups characterize aerobic exercise.

If you are exercising at a pace that is too intense, your body will utilize the *anaerobic* energy system. This type of exercise quickly uses up more oxygen than the body can take in while engaging in the exercise, causing an oxygen debt. This, in turn, causes lactic acids (waste products) to accumulate in the muscles, which leads to exhaustion.

Anaerobic activity is basically stop and start, in which the heart is *not* kept at a constant, steady pace for 20 to 60 minutes. Thus, anaerobic describes an activity that requires all-out effort of short duration and does not utilize oxygen to produce energy.

By engaging in step training or any other aerobic activity, the heart gradually strengthens and develops a greater capacity to pump more oxygenated blood to the body with fewer contractions. Exercised hearts are stronger and slower.

> Highly trained and conditioned endurance athletes have resting heart rates as low as 30 to 32 beats per minute, an unbelievably low rate! What happens is that, with regular, stimulating exercise, the heart becomes a more efficient pump. It pumps more blood with each stroke, and with a more efficient stroke volume, your heart can function with less effort.
>
> By getting your heart into condition, you may be practicing preventive medicine. You may be lessening the danger of a coronary heart attack, 5, 10, 15, 20 years from now. And if you do have a heart attack, your chances of surviving are far greater with a heart, lungs, and blood vessels that are in good condition.[3]

A person can exist without big, bulging muscles, or without the perfect figure, or with a head cold, but not very long without a good heart and lungs. Unfortunately, more than 40% of all people who have a first heart attack do not have a second chance to change their habits or develop an aerobic program. They die. And more than half of all deaths in the United States each year are attributable to heart-related diseases.[4] If only we could establish a priority early in life to counteract this overwhelming statistic!

## Flexibility

Flexibility is defined as *the functional range of motion of a certain joint and its corresponding muscle groups.* The greater the range of movement, the more the muscles, tendons, and ligaments can flex or bend.

Muscles are arranged in pairs. One muscle's ability to shorten or contract is directly related to the opposing muscle's length or stretch. Flexibility is maintained or increased by movement patterns that slowly and progressively stretch the muscle beyond its relaxed length. The stretch is performed to a point at which the exerciser feels tension developing in the muscle, but not to a point of pain.

## Muscular Strength and Endurance

Muscular strength is the *ability of a muscle to exert a force against a resistance.* Strength activities increase the amount of force muscles can exert, or the amount of work muscles can perform. Activities such as weight training can develop strength in the skeletal muscles.

Muscular endurance is the *ability of muscles to work strenuously for relatively long periods without fatigue.* It is the capacity of a muscle to exert a force repeatedly, or to hold a static (still) contraction over time.

Muscular strength and endurance activities do not provide increased oxygen to condition the heart to function more efficiently.[5] Their primary target is skeletal muscle.

## Good Posture/Good Positioning

Proper positioning of the body when performing any type of physical exertion promotes a safe and efficient workout. Once the basic mechanics are known and practiced, this underlying fitness component becomes an integral part of every move, not a separate program.

## Body Composition

An individual's total body weight is composed of fat weight and lean weight (fat-free weight). Keeping an appropriate percentage ratio between these two weights is important for the entire body's best functioning and helps prevent obesity and its many related health risks. This fitness component is managed by establishing a proper diet and exercise plan that provides for maintaining ideal weight.

If you aren't beginning your program at an ideal weight, specific guidelines will be given within both the physical exercise programs and the dietary eating plans you'll establish for how to achieve an ideal percentage ratio.

## ◼ Aerobic Fitness Training

The remainder of Chapter 1 is devoted to a detailed look at aerobic fitness research and the general principles recommended for you to follow, including modes of activity to choose in addition to step training. The other four physical fitness components are explained more fully in later chapters.

Aerobic means promoting the supply and use of oxygen, and training refers to muscle stimulation. Therefore, aerobic training is any exercise that requires a steady supply of oxygen for an extended time and demands an uninterrupted work output from the muscles.

An activity such as step training significantly increases the oxygen supply to all body parts, including the heart and lungs, through continuous, rhythmic movement of large muscles and connective tissue. This type of movement conditions the body's oxygen transport system (heart, lungs, blood, and blood vessels) to process oxygen more efficiently. This *efficiency in processing oxygen,* called *aerobic capacity,* is dependent on your ability to:

◼ Rapidly breathe large amounts of air.

◼ Forcefully deliver large volumes of blood.

◼ Effectively deliver oxygen to all parts of the body.

In short, one's aerobic capacity depends upon efficient lungs, a powerful heart, and a good vascular system. Because it reflects the conditions of these vital organs, *aerobic capacity is the best index (single measure) of overall physical fitness.*[6]

Aerobic capacity is what is measured, quantified, and labeled in a physical fitness stress test, performed either in a laboratory (called a laboratory stress test) or on a premeasured distance such as a track (called a field stress test). Chapter 2 describes these and other ways by which you can test your aerobic capacity.

## The Progressive Overload Principle

Step training, or any aerobic activity, conditions the heart muscle by strengthening it through a principle called *progressive overload.* Not only will the heart pump more blood with each beat, but it will also rest longer between each beat, thereby lowering the pulse rate.

Aerobic exercise overloads the heart by causing it to beat faster during the specific timeframe of the workout session, producing a temporary high demand on the cardiorespiratory system. Over time, as you become more fit, the heart eventually will adjust to this temporary high demand, and soon it will be able to do the same amount of work with less effort.

By overloading the heart with any vigorous aerobic exercise, your aerobic capacity will increase and you can achieve a desirable training effect. The *training effect,* or total beneficial changes that usually occur, consists of the following:

◼ Stronger heart, sending more oxygenated blood to all tissues of the body.

◼ More blood cells produced.

◼ Slower resting heart rate.

- Expansion of blood vessels.
- Improvement in muscle tone.
- Lower blood pressure through improved circulation.
- Stronger respiratory muscles.
- Regulation of the release of adrenalin.
- Greater lung capacity.
- More regular elimination of solid wastes.
- Lower levels of fat in blood.[7]
- Strengthening of muscles and skeleton to protect them from injury later in life.
- Increased bone density, deterring osteoporosis.[8]
- Increased sensitivity to insulin and lowered blood sugar levels in mild, adult-onset diabetes.[9]
- Improvement in the way the body handles cholesterol, by increasing the proportion of blood cholesterol attached to high-density lipoprotein — a carrier molecule that keeps cholesterol from damaging artery walls.[10]

## Alternative Aerobic Exercise

In addition to bench/step training, aerobic exercise options include all of the following activities:

- Aerobic dance-exercise (aerobics)
- Cross-country skiing
- Cycling (including stationary cycling)

- Jogging/running
- Jumping rope
- Rowing
- Skating (ice/roller/in-line)
- Stair climbing
- Swimming
- Walking/hiking (moderate to fast pace-walk).

## Aerobic Criteria

These exercise alternatives, collectively, must have several essential criteria for the exercise to be labeled *aerobic* (see Figure 1.1). Because aerobic means *with oxygen*:

1. *The movement you do must use the large muscles of the body,*[11] (arms and legs). The gesture and step patterns in bench/step movements are excellent choices.

2. *The movement must be rhythmic.*[12] One-two-one-two, using a steady beat of music, with either a fast or slow tempo, is suggested.

3. *You must practice a minimum of three sessions per week.*[13]

   - 4 days a week or every other day is good.
   - Some key researchers recommend 5 days as a maximum for fitness goals. Beyond this, injuries to the musculoskeletal system from

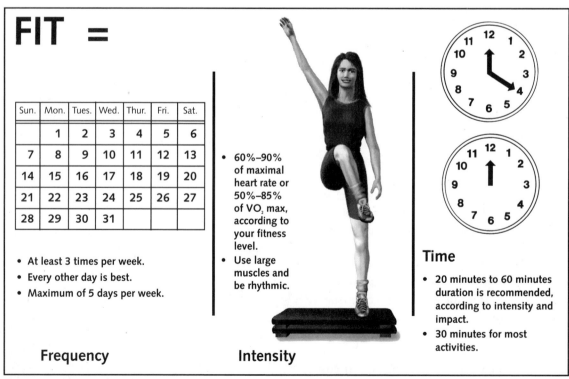

| Sun. | Mon. | Tues. | Wed. | Thur. | Fri. | Sat. |
|------|------|-------|------|-------|------|------|
|      | 1    | 2     | 3    | 4     | 5    | 6    |
| 7    | 8    | 9     | 10   | 11    | 12   | 13   |
| 14   | 15   | 16    | 17   | 18    | 19   | 20   |
| 21   | 22   | 23    | 24   | 25    | 26   | 27   |
| 28   | 29   | 30    | 31   |       |      |      |

**Frequency**
- At least 3 times per week.
- Every other day is best.
- Maximum of 5 days per week.

**Intensity**
- 60%–90% of maximal heart rate or 50%–85% of VO$_2$ max, according to your fitness level.
- Use large muscles and be rhythmic.

**Time**
- 20 minutes to 60 minutes duration is recommended, according to intensity and impact.
- 30 minutes for most activities.

**Figure 1.1.** Five aerobic criteria.

overuse are 10 times more likely to occur. Give your body at least 2 days off per week, especially if you are a novice to physical fitness conditioning.

- If your goals are related to more than just aerobic fitness — if, perhaps, your profession (such as a fitness instructor) or your athletic sport status requires more workouts or days per week — allow your body to tell you your maximum frequency. A sudden elevated resting heart rate in the morning signifies the day(s) not to work out. This is your built-in body signal, and it can be readily seen/ heard/felt simply by daily monitoring your resting heart rate. Upon arising in the morning, check this heart rate for 1 full minute.

4. *You must exercise continuously for 20–60 minutes.*[14]

- Duration depends upon the intensity used, and the impact of the activity.
- Lower intensity activity, such as walking, should be done over a longer period (40–60 minutes).
- Because high-impact types of activity, such as running and jumping, generally cause significantly more debilitating injuries to exercisers, shorter workouts (20 minutes) are recommended.

5. To receive the cardiorespiratory fitness benefits (called the training effect), *the heart rate must be maintained in a specific target heart rate training zone*, which is the individualized safe pace at which to aerobically work or exercise. This reflects your intensity and is explained scientifically as one of the following:

- 60% to 90% of your maximum heart rate, *or*
- 50% to 85% of your maximum oxygen uptake, or heart rate reserve.[15]

## Intensity

Frequency and time duration of your workouts are easy to determine. Determining the amount of exertion during the workout to keep it safe while continually making fitness gains can

be more of a challenge, especially for the novice. Intensity is measured (monitored) in one of three ways:

- Finding your *target heart rate (THR)* training zone using the Karvonen formula. This is suggested for the novice.
- Using the psychophysical scale for *ratings of perceived exertion (RPE)*, which shows a high correlation with heart rate and other metabolic parameters, according to American College of Sports Medicine (ACSM) guidelines. Rate of perceived exertion monitoring is suggested for the individual who already has become well-accustomed to taking a heart rate pulse.
- Using the *talk test*. This easy and practical method is best used in conjunction with the THR and RPE for monitoring exercise intensity.

## TARGET HEART RATE

**Taking Your Pulse.** To calculate appropriate exercise intensity by finding your THR training zone, you first must know how to accurately take your pulse. The pulse equals heartbeats per minute and can be felt and counted at one of six pulsation points. Select which area you can best obtain a pulse using your index and second fingers. The two places most often used to count pulse are the neck near the carotid artery and the wrist near the radial artery. Both are shown in Figure 1.2.

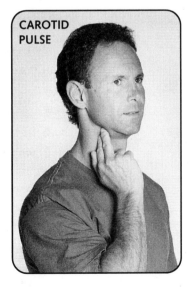
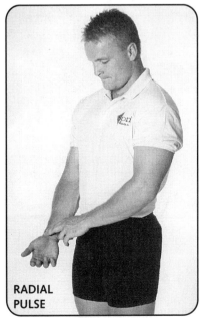

**Figure 1.2.** Taking the pulse at the carotid artery and the radial artery.

1. The *carotid artery*, located in the neck, is usually easy to find. Place your index and middle fingers below the point of your jawbone and slide downward an inch or so, pressing lightly. When you use the carotid artery method, make sure to apply light pressure, as excessive pressure may cause the heart rate to slow down by a reflex action.

2. The *radial artery* extends up the wrist on the thumb side. Place your index and middle fingers just below the base of your thumb. Press lightly. Count the number of pulsations, or beats, for 60 seconds. The total is the number of heartbeats per minute. To count correctly, make sure you count each beat you feel.

Having gained the skill of pulse taking, it is now time to establish your *resting heart rate*. This number is to be placed in the formula for establishing your target heart rate training zone.

**Establishing Resting Heart Rate (RHR).** A true *resting* heart rate (RHR) is not taken in a class but, instead, when the individual has been at complete rest, preferably after sleeping for several hours and upon awakening. Keep a clock or watch with a second hand next to your bed. When you awaken (without an alarm clock ring), take your pulse for 1 full minute and record that number as your RHR. Do this for five consecutive mornings, then determine an average (add all RHR's and divide by 5). This is a rather accurate way to determine your resting heart rate.

---

**WEEK 1:**

Day 1: _____

Day 2: _____

Day 3: _____

Day 4: _____

Day 5: _____

Sum total: _____

÷ 5: _____ RHR

---

> *Unusual stress and illness (illness is a type of stress) sharply elevate the resting heart rate from previous readings.*

Normally healthy individuals should find a positive outlet for stress. Stress affects you even as you sleep. The heart continues to beat rapidly at a time when the heart ideally should take a break and slow down for 6 to 8 hours.

One of the two visible signs of improvement in heart and lung fitness is a lower resting heart rate. Because the RHR is the basic thermometer of fitness, after a 10-to-15-week step aerobics course, you and your classmates may experience:

■ A decline in your resting heart rate beats per minute.

■ A significant decline in resting heart rate beats per minute by smokers who quit, or cut down their intake, during the course.

Continue to monitor and record your RHR at least two times per week in a Fitness Journal you keep for the course.

**Determining THR Training Zone.** You can now place your average RHR figure in the formula for determining your target heart rate training zone, in Table 1.1. The other variables figured into the formula are your current *age* and *lifestyle*, represented as a percentage of your maximum heart rate.

In Table 1.1, record your current age and the percentage range you select from the list below that describes your current lifestyle.

| If you are: | Use: |
|---|---|
| ■ a nonathletic adult | 50% to begin |
| ■ sedentary | 60%-69% |
| ■ moderately active | 70%-75% |
| ■ very active and well-trained | 80%-85% |

Now figure the Karvonen equation. The result is your target heart rate training zone, the safe exercise training zone for you.

**Taking a Count After a Step Aerobics Interval.** As you are beginning a step aerobics program, you will want to monitor your pace several times during the workout hour so you can learn constant endurance pacing. Mentally remember your

## TABLE 1.1    How to Figure Your Target Heart Rate Training Zone

The following three basic factors enter into figuring your estimated safe exercise zone.

1.  Your current age: _____

2.  How active is your lifestyle? _____    _____% MHR.

If you are:

> *(Choose one:)*
>
> ▮ Nonathletic adult: use 50% of your maximum heart rate.
> ▮ Sedentary: use the figure 60%–69% of your maximum heart rate (but only for the first 2 or 3 weeks).
> ▮ Moderately physically active: use 70–75% of your maximum heart rate.
> ▮ Active and well-trained: use 80–85% of your maximum heart rate.

3.  Your average resting heart rate: (see page 8):_____

Now place your numbers in the Karvonen formula, which follows:

A.  220 _____ − _____ = _____ **Estimated Maximal Heart Rate (MHR)**
    **(Index number)**        **(Your Age)**

B.  _____ − _____ = _____
    **MHR**              **Resting HR**              **HR Reserve**

C.  _____ × . _____ = _____ + **Resting HR** = _____ *
    **Heart Rate Reserve**        **Lower end lifestyle activity range**
                                  **(#2 above)**

    _____ × . _____ = _____ + **Resting HR** = _____ *
    **Heart Rate Reserve**        **Higher end lifestyle activity range**
                                  **(#2 above)**

**RANGE**

**RANGE OF**     _____ *     This range is your estimated safe exercise zone. Keep your heart rate
**YOUR**                               working in this range while you exercise aerobically for approximately 30
**TARGET**       _____ *     minutes of each session.

                                       Refigure as you "age," as you can reclassify your lifestyle of activity, or as
                                       your resting heart rate markedly declines.

Example: Chris is 20 years old, a moderately active person (70%–75% range), with a resting heart rate of 62.

A.  220 − 20 = 200 MHR

B.  200 − 62 = 138 Heart Rate Reserve

C.  138 × .70 =   96 + 62 = 158*     Target Heart Rate Training Zone
    138 × .75 = 104 + 62 = 166*

If Chris keeps working (aerobically exercising) at the range of 158 to 166 heartbeats per minute, the heart will be safely working toward the training effect.

readings, and record them at the end of each class in your Fitness Journal.

When you take a pulse rate during the learning process and find that your pace is *below* your established training zone, *increase* your intensity. If you have a pulse rate *higher* than your established training zone, *lower* your intensity.

To become familiar with your own response to various intensity levels so you can better regulate yourself, ask yourself, "How do I feel when I get this pulse?" Focus not only on your pulse count but also on what feelings and conditions the number relates to, so you can begin to recognize the signals your body sends.

This also will help prepare you to use the RPE monitoring method of intensity, which, as you become a more advanced exerciser, will be a more practical and practiced method than counting your heartbeats per minute.

If you are working above your training zone, you are working anaerobically and will not be able to sustain the activity for a long time. Monitor your intensity and adjust your workout accordingly. Slow down, walk around, find your pulse, and count it for either 6 *or* 10 seconds. Each of these counts has been found to be a scientifically accurate measurement for aerobic activity pulse rates. Taking a timed count of greater than 10 seconds immediately after aerobic exercise will tend to be inaccurate because the heart rate slows to a recovery pulse rapidly. You or your instructor will determine whether you will count for 6 or 10 seconds.

**6-Second Count Method:** Immediately following the step aerobic exercise segment, count your pulse and multiply the number you get times 10. This newly multiplied number will equal heartbeats per minute and hopefully will always be in your safe training zone.

> *Taking a 6-second count is easy. All you do is add a zero to the pulse you feel, and record that number. You must carefully begin and end exactly with a timer.*

**10-Second Count Method:** Count your pulse for 10 seconds immediately following the step aerobic exercise segment, and multiply the number you get times 6. This newly multiplied number will equal heartbeats per minute and should be in the safe exercise training zone you established for yourself.

For ease in figuring the 10-second count, Table 1.2 lists target heart rate counts for individuals who wish to attain fitness using the ideal aerobic range for most people (60%–75% of heart rate reserve). Locate the column across the top that is closest to your age and the row down the left side reflecting a figure closest to your resting heart rate. The box where the column and row intersect is *your 10-second target heart rate training zone.* The numbers in the squares represent pulse beats counted in 10 seconds.

As your cardiovascular and respiratory systems become more fit and efficient, exercise will become easier, and you will have to increase the intensity of your activities. Techniques for increasing and decreasing the intensity of your workout will be explained later. By using the target heart rate training zone, you automatically compensate for increased fitness and still maintain the same training effect.

Thus, your heart rate increases during the vigorous aerobic step training activity and should return to normal (pre-activity heart rate) within a

**TABLE 1.2    Target Heart Rate Training Zones Using 10-Second Count Method**

| Your Average Resting Heart Rate ▼ | 15 | 20 | 25 | 30 | 35 | 40 | 45 | 50 | 55 | 60 | 65 | 70 | 75 | 80 |
|---|---|---|---|---|---|---|---|---|---|---|---|---|---|---|
| 90 | 27-29 | 26-29 | 26-28 | 25-28 | 25-27 | 24-26 | 23-26 | 23-25 | 22-24 | 22-24 | 21-23 | 21-22 | 20-22 | 20-21 |
| 85 | 26-29 | 26-29 | 25-28 | 25-27 | 24-27 | 24-26 | 23-25 | 23-25 | 22-24 | 22-24 | 21-23 | 21-22 | 20-22 | 20-21 |
| 80 | 26-29 | 25-28 | 25-28 | 24-27 | 24-26 | 23-26 | 23-25 | 22-25 | 22-24 | 21-23 | 21-23 | 20-22 | 20-21 | 19-21 |
| 75 | 26-29 | 25-28 | 25-28 | 24-27 | 24-26 | 23-26 | 23-25 | 22-25 | 21-24 | 21-23 | 20-23 | 20-22 | 19-21 | 19-21 |
| 70 | 25-29 | 25-28 | 24-27 | 24-27 | 23-26 | 23-25 | 22-25 | 22-24 | 21-24 | 21-24 | 20-22 | 20-22 | 19-21 | 19-20 |
| 65 | 25-28 | 25-28 | 24-27 | 23-26 | 23-26 | 22-25 | 21-24 | 21-23 | 20-23 | 20-22 | 19-21 | 19-21 | 18-20 |
| 60 | 25-28 | 24-28 | 24-27 | 23-26 | 23-26 | 22-25 | 21-24 | 21-24 | 20-23 | 20-22 | 19-22 | 19-21 | 18-21 | 18-20 |
| 55 | 24-27 | 23-27 | 23-27 | 23-26 | 22-25 | 21-24 | 21-24 | 21-24 | 20-23 | 20-22 | 19-22 | 19-21 | 18-20 | 18-20 |
| 50 | 24-28 | 23-27 | 23-26 | 22-26 | 22-25 | 21-25 | 21-24 | 20-23 | 20-23 | 19-22 | 19-21 | 18-21 | 18-20 | 17-20 |

short time after the workout. As a rule, the faster it slows down (recovers from exercise), the more physically fit you are, as recovery heart rate improvement is another indication of an increased fitness level.

## RPE USING THE BORG SCALE

The second method for monitoring intensity utilizes the psychophysical Borg scale for ratings of perceived exertion (RPE),[16] as shown in Table 1.3. This scale is based on the finding that, while exercising, one has the ability to accurately assess how hard the body is working. It is basically a judgment call and is more appropriate when used by individuals who have been exercising for some time. The untrained exerciser typically reports a higher RPE than an athlete, at the same exercise heart rate.

RPE seems to correlate strongly with other workload indicators, such as ventilation, oxygen consumption, and muscle metabolism. Participants tune into the overall sensation of effort exerted by their entire body, rather than one factor such as local calf or hamstring exhaustion, panting, sweating, or body temperature. When used along with heart rate monitoring, RPE is useful for the novice, who may not yet be aware of how exercise is supposed to feel.

You might begin to make mental notes to yourself during the workout hour concerning your ratings of perceived exertion. After the workout, immediately record what you felt for each phase of the workout, expressed as numbers from 0 to 10. Begin to notice the correlation between target heart rates you achieve and how ratings of perceived exertion feel.

## TALK TEST

A third and less formal method for determining aerobic intensity is called the *talk test*. It is based on the premise that, while exercising, the participant should always be able to maintain a conversation. If the participant can gasp out only one or

### TABLE 1.3 Borg Scale Ratings of Perceived Exertion

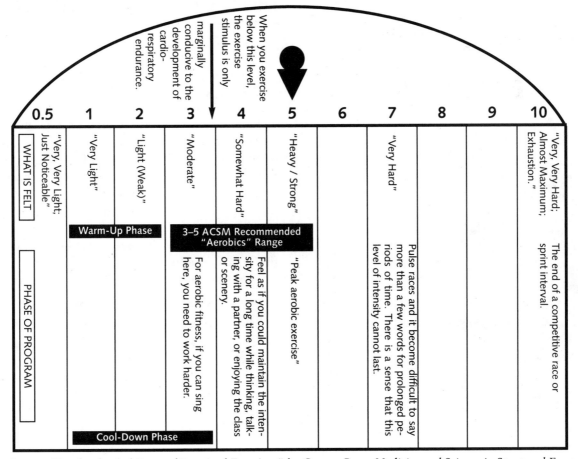

Source: "Psychophysical Bases of Perceived Exertion," by Gunnar Borg, *Medicine and Science in Sport and Exercise* 14 (1982).

two words at a time, the exercise intensity is probably anaerobic and should be adjusted to allow for two- to three-word phrases. Because the accuracy of the talk test varies within any given population, it is best utilized in conjunction with the THR and the RPE for monitoring exercise intensity.[17]

### WHICH METHOD IS BEST?

The experts do not agree when it comes to THR versus RPE. Some claim that only THR methods are accurate; others believe that RPE and the talk test are more practical. Because all the methods are useful and none is consistently ideal, a good solution is to *use a combination of all three*. Once a participant has developed a good understanding of the heart rate/RPE relationship, heart rate can be monitored less frequently and RPE can be used as a primary means of measuring exercise intensity with the talk test as an informal supplemental backup measure.[18]

## ▌ Total Physical Fitness: A Choice

*Physical Activity and Health: A Report of the Surgeon General* compiled data collected from years of research examining the effects of physical activity on health. The research indicates that regular physical activity can improve one's health and wellness. The report also reveals that more than 60% of adults do not achieve the recommended amount of physical activity and 25% of adults do not exercise at all. The Surgeon General's policy statement — that 30 minutes of regular physical activity of moderate intensity done on most days of the week — is one of the best things you can do for your health.[19] Major findings include the following:

▌ People who are inactive can improve their health and wellness by being moderately active on a regular basis.

▌ Physical activity does not have to be strenuous to achieve health benefits.

▌ Moderate-intensity physical activity has significant health benefits, and vigorous physical activity has an even greater health benefit.

If you are beginning an exercise program, the Surgeon General's findings should encourage you to get started. Even a little bit of activity will be a step in your journey to becoming physically fit.

### SUMMARY

Achieving physical fitness requires dedication to personal excellence. There are few shortcuts but many pleasurable alternatives. Once achieved, you must continue to make choices that maintain your fitness for a lifetime. Fitness is a journey — a continual process — not just one destination. Maintaining fitness is a lot easier than initially achieving it, though you will discover that the less physically fit you are, the longer you will take to become fit.

The total physical fitness journey requires:

▌ Seeking safe, valid information.

▌ Establishing your starting points.

▌ Setting reasonable and challenging goals.

▌ Monitoring your daily progress.

▌ Continually making self-disciplined choices.

Enjoy the journey!

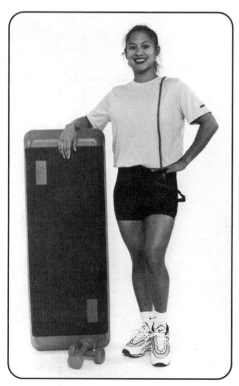

Physical fitness is the positive state of well-being.

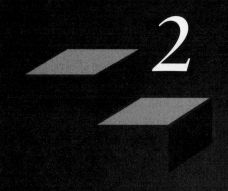

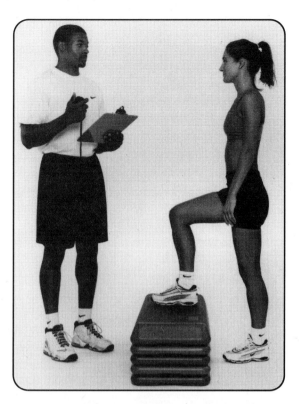

# THE FIRST STEP: DETERMINING YOUR STARTING POINT

The first step in the journey toward achieving, and then maintaining, physical fitness for a lifetime involves establishing your current fitness starting points, using scientific prescreening, test and assessment procedures. Clearly knowing yourself in terms of your past history, risk factors, and present physical status will assist you in developing a lifetime fitness plan. It will enable you to realistically and safely set achievable short-term fitness goals. It also will provide the basis for continually motivating you to adhere to the program you do establish, to achieve your long-range and lifetime fitness goals.

It can be painful and devastating to realize you are out of shape and test poorly on laboratory or field stress tests. No one wants to see scientific results that label him or her inferior or below the norm. It takes determination and courage to find out just where you are at the outset. Then, with time and dedication, it is motivating to progress to the point where your post-assessment test numbers represent an excellent state of total fitness and well-being.

In most instances, specific fitness testing is appropriate only after obtaining a medical history. Prescreening may uncover potential problems and determine if you should be considered for a specific exercise prescription. Most course settings require this prescreening — or a thorough medical exam if you have any limitations or known risk factors.

## Principles of Fitness Assessments

The purpose of an initial pre-course fitness assessment is to *establish a baseline of information from which later changes can be compared.* Assessment principles include the following:

1. Testing is an effective way to measure *improvement* in performance over time, and not as an absolutely correct physiologic measurement or comparison.

2. By following consistent procedures of testing (using the same test, the same person administering it, and the same time of day), you are more assured of accuracy in measurement over time.

3. Results are recorded for comparison purposes. The person being tested should understand these values and ask questions as needed to ensure understanding.

## Measuring Aerobic Capacity

Pre-assessing your current status by having a thorough physical fitness exam will measure your heart's response to increasing amounts of exercise, or ability to use oxygen. Physical fitness should be measured in one of two ways at least every 3 years:

1. A laboratory physical fitness test.
2. A field test administered by you and a friend.

### The Laboratory Physical Fitness Test

The key to good health and exercising without fear is a properly conducted treadmill stress test to check out the precise condition of your heart.[1] Physical fitness and health are different, and the treadmill stress ECG helps to make that distinction.[2]

Prior to a treadmill stress test, you will be thoroughly screened. This consists of:

1. A brief history-taking and physical exam, during which the technician listens to your heart and lungs

2. A check for the use of drugs known to affect the ECG (various heart and hypertensive medications)

3. A check for history of congenital or acquired heart disorders

4. An evaluation of the resting ECG.

This screening and background check will help to determine your risk factors. A *risk factor* is a feature in a person's heredity, background, or present lifestyle that increases the likelihood of developing coronary heart disease. If no risk factors are present, an exercise test usually is not necessary below age 35 if you follow the guidelines mentioned earlier. If symptoms of heart, lung, or metabolic disease are present, a maximum stress test is recommended for individuals of any age prior to the onset of a vigorous exercise program, and followed with tests every 2 years.[3]

### SUB-MAXIMAL TESTING

Sub-maximal testing is accomplished by means of a physical fitness test (stress test) on a treadmill. Electrocardiogram leads transmit and record electrical heart impulses that are read on a machine and recorded on a strip of paper, called an electrocardiograph. You are tested only to approximately 150 beats per minute, not to exhaustion.

The ECG electrodes with leads are circular rubber discs with wires attached to them. The discs are glued onto the chest and back at key locations so various "pictures" of your heart, from different angles and sides, can all be recorded at once. Usually between seven and 10 electrodes are applied, depending on the laboratory's procedures or the individual's specific needs.

You probably will be asked to walk at a pace of 3.3 miles per hour (90 meters per minute) on the treadmill. The grade will begin flat and will increase slowly in gradation, as if you were walking up a hill. Every minute the "hill" will become steeper and more difficult to climb.

When your heart rate reaches 150 beats per minute, a record is made of the amount of time it took you to arrive at that reading. Then, through an indirect method of extrapolation (projection of maximum results from having tested many others the same way in the past), your fitness ability is estimated.

Basically, the longer your heart rate takes to reach 150 beats per minute, the more fit you are; the shorter, the less fit you are. Sub-maximal fitness testing usually is done with those who know of no outstanding limitations and who are interested in starting an aerobic step training program.

### MAXIMAL TESTING

Maximal testing procedures are administered if an individual has a more specific need. Maximum testing directly reveals how much oxygen you use, because you are tested to exhaustion. The exhaustion point is when you start to get markedly fatigued. Some researchers believe that maximum laboratory testing is the *only* conclusive type to use.

## Field Tests of Aerobic Fitness

You may not have immediate access to a laboratory and qualified physiologists to monitor the results recorded with the treadmill method. Therefore, field tests have been developed to help you assess your own physical fitness by determining your current aerobic capacity. This testing is easily conducted in an aerobics class setting.

The information and Tables 2.1 and 2.2 were developed from Dr. Kenneth Cooper's book, *The*

*If you are over age 35, you should start an aerobic step training program by first seeing your doctor and then taking a monitored laboratory fitness test. Individuals with known cardiovascular, pulmonary, or metabolic disease should have a maximum stress test prior to beginning vigorous exercise at any age. These people and those whose exercise tests are abnormal should get a stress test annually.*

### TABLE 2.1    Cooper's 12-Minute Walking/Running Test: Distance (Miles) Covered

| Fitness Category | | Age (years) 13-19 | 20-29 | 30-39 | 40-49 | 50-59 | 60 + |
|---|---|---|---|---|---|---|---|
| I. Very Poor | (men) | <1.30 | <1.22 | <1.18 | <1.14 | <1.03 | < .87 |
| | (women) | < 1.0 | < .96 | < .94 | < .88 | < .84 | < .78 |
| II. Poor | (men) | 1.30-1.37 | 1.22-1.31 | 1.18-1.30 | 1.14-1.24 | 1.03-1.16 | .87-1.02 |
| | (women) | 1.00-1.18 | .96-1.11 | .95-1.05 | .88- .98 | .84- .93 | .78- .86 |
| III. Fair | (men) | 1.38-1.56 | 1.32-1.49 | 1.31-1.45 | 1.25-1.39 | 1.17-1.30 | 1.03-1.20 |
| | (women) | 1.19-1.29 | 1.12-1.22 | 1.06-1.18 | .99-1.11 | .94-1.05 | .87- .98 |
| IV. Good | (men) | 1.57-1.72 | 1.50-1.64 | 1.46-1.56 | 1.40-1.53 | 1.31-1.44 | 1.21-1.32 |
| | (women) | 1.30-1.43 | 1.23-1.34 | 1.19-1.29 | 1.12-1.24 | 1.06-1.18 | .99-1.09 |
| V. Excellent | (men) | 1.73-1.86 | 1.65-1.76 | 1.57-1.69 | 1.54-1.65 | 1.45-1.58 | 1.33-1.55 |
| | (women) | 1.44-1.51 | 1.35-1.45 | 1.30-1.39 | 1.25-1.34 | 1.19-1.30 | 1.10-1.18 |
| VI. Superior | (men) | >1.87 | >1.77 | >1.70 | >1.66 | >1.59 | >1.56 |
| | (women) | >1.52 | >1.46 | >1.40 | >1.35 | >1.31 | >1.19 |

< Means less than; > more than.

From *The Aerobics Program For Total Well-Being*, by Kenneth H. Cooper, M.D., M.P.H., Copyright ©1982 by Kenneth H. Cooper. Reprinted by permission of the publisher, Bantam-Doubleday-Dell, New York, NY 10103.

### PRE-TEST:

Start Time: _____        Stop Time: _____        Distance Covered: _____

Check for your Fitness Category, above in Table 2.1.

**Circle Fitness Category:**    Very Poor / Poor / Fair / Good / Excellent / Superior    **COURSE GOAL:** _____

### POST-TEST:

Start Time: _____        Stop Time: _____        Distance Covered: _____

Check for your Fitness Category, above in Table 2.1.

**Circle Fitness Category:**    Very Poor / Poor / Fair / Good / Excellent / Superior    **2-MONTH GOAL:** _____

**TABLE 2.2    Cooper's 1.5-Mile Run/Walk Test: Time (Minutes)**

| | | Age (years) | | | | | |
| --- | --- | --- | --- | --- | --- | --- | --- |
| **Fitness Category** | | **13-19** | **20-29** | **30-39** | **40-49** | **50-59** | **60 +** |
| I. Very Poor | (men) | >15:31 | >16:01 | >16:31 | >17:31 | >19:01 | >20:01 |
| | (women) | >18:31 | >19:01 | >19:31 | >20:01 | >20:31 | >21:01 |
| II. Poor | (men) | 12:11-15:30 | 14:01-16:00 | 14:44-16:30 | 15:36-17:30 | 17:01-19:00 | 19:01-20:00 |
| | (women) | 16:55-18:30 | 18:31-19:00 | 19:01-19:30 | 19:31-20:00 | 20:01-20:30 | 21:00-21:31 |
| III. Fair | (men) | 10:49-12:10 | 12:01-14:00 | 12:31-14:45 | 13:01-15:35 | 14:31-17:00 | 16:16-19:00 |
| | (women) | 14:31-16:54 | 15:55-18:30 | 16:31-19:00 | 17:31-19:30 | 19:01-20:00 | 19:31-20:30 |
| IV. Good | (men) | 9:41-10:48 | 10:46-12:00 | 11:01-12:30 | 11:31-13:00 | 12:31-14:30 | 14:00-16:15 |
| | (women) | 12:30-14:30 | 13:31-15:54 | 14:31-16:30 | 15:56-17:30 | 16:31-19:00 | 17:31-19:30 |
| V. Excellent | (men) | 8:37- 9:40 | 9:45-10:45 | 10:00-11:00 | 10:30-11:30 | 11:00-12:30 | 11:15-13:59 |
| | (women) | 11:50-12:29 | 12:30-13:30 | 13:00-14:30 | 13:45-15:55 | 14:30-16:30 | 16:30-17:30 |
| VI. Superior | (men) | < 8:37 | < 9:45 | <10:00 | <10:30 | <11:00 | <11:15 |
| | (women) | <11:50 | <12:30 | <13:00 | <13:45 | <14:30 | <16:30 |

< Means less than; > more than.

From *The Aerobics Program For Total Well-Being*, by Kenneth H. Cooper, M.D., M.P.H., Copyright ©1982 by Kenneth H. Cooper. Reprinted by permission of the publisher, Bantam-Doubleday-Dell, New York, NY 10103.

## PRE-TEST:

Check Off Laps: (i.e., 14 for 190-yd. track; 21 for 126-yd. track):

1 - 2 - 3 - 4 - 5 - 6 - 7 - 8 - 9 - 10 - 11 - 12 - 13 - 14 - 15 - 16 - 17 - 18 - 19 - 20 - 21

Time: _____ OR: Just record here if using an open roadway.

Stop Time: _____

–Start Time: _____

Time: _____

Check for your Fitness Category, above in Table 2.2.

**Circle Fitness Category:**   Very Poor / Poor / Fair / Good / Excellent / Superior   **COURSE GOAL:** _____

## POST-TEST:

Check Off Laps: (i.e., 14 for 190-yd. track; 21 for 126-yd. track):

1 - 2 - 3 - 4 - 5 - 6 - 7 - 8 - 9 - 10 - 11 - 12 - 13 - 14 - 15 - 16 - 17 - 18 - 19 - 20 - 21

Time: _____ OR: Just record here if using an open roadway.

Stop Time: _____

–Start Time: _____

Time: _____

Check for your Fitness Category, above in Table 2.2.

**Circle Fitness Category:**   Very Poor / Poor / Fair / Good / Excellent / Superior   **2-MONTH GOAL:** _____

*Aerobics Program for Total Well-Being.*[4] Cooper's 12-Minute Test and 1.5 Mile Test are two that you can administer by yourself or with the help of a friend.

As guidelines for field testing:

1. If you previously have been physically inactive, participate in 1 to 2 weeks of walking or beginning step aerobics before undertaking either of Cooper's tests.

2. Wear loose clothing in which you can freely sweat, and a sport shoe (such as a "cross-trainer").

3. Determine first which field test you plan to take. You can choose running with time or distance as the stopping point.

   ▪ If *time* is the stopping point, take the 12-minute test.

   ▪ If *distance* is the stopping point, take the 1.5-mile test.

   ▪ If you believe that you are really out of shape, *the 12-minute test will be easier* because you run for this amount of time only. (An individual might take 20 minutes to complete 1.5 miles.)

4. Be sure you have a stopwatch or a second hand on your watch, or that you are close to a wall timer.

5. Immediately before performing the test, spend 5 to 10 minutes warming up the muscles (see Chapter 4).

6. Have a partner record your data (as time it takes, or laps, or distance).

7. Run or walk (or a combination) as quickly as you can for 12 minutes or 1.5 miles (see Figure 2.1). This is an all-out test of endurance.

8. When you stop, identify precisely the *distance* covered in miles and tenths of miles or *time* it took, and have your partner record it on Table 2.1 or Table 2.2.

9. Cool down by first walking slowly for several minutes, and finish by doing cool-down stretching.

10. Interpret and record, on Tables 2.1 or 2.2, your results for the specific test you used. Reassess your fitness at the end of the course. How did you change from the pre-test to the post-test?

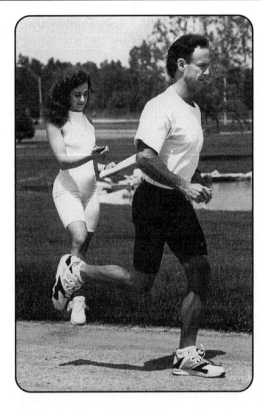

**Figure 2.1** Run or walk as quickly as you can for 12 minutes or 1.5 miles.

## 3-Minute Step Test for Aerobic Capacity

Another method used to determine cardiovascular endurance or aerobic capacity is the 3-Minute Step Test, developed by Dr. Fred Kasch, San Diego. The YMCA uses it for testing a large group of participants. Although this method is easy to administer and requires little equipment, the American Council on Exercise notes the inconsistency of the results when compared to other methods for determining aerobic capacity.[5]

Before taking the 3-Minute Step Test, be certain that you can accurately monitor your pulse (see Chapter 1). Once you have developed this skill you are ready to take this easy-to-perform test. You will need a 12" step, a timepiece, and a metronome (or music) at a tempo of 96 beats per minute (bpm).

1. Before you begin, warm up for a few minutes by walking or performing another low-intensity exercise for 5 to 10 minutes to gradually increase the heart rate and warm up the muscles. Light stretching may also be helpful.

2. To perform the test, step onto and off the 12" step platform to the cadence of the metronome or music set at 96 counts per minute.

3. The step pattern is a simple four-count cycle: Step *up right*, step *up left*, step *down right* and step *down left*, for 3 minutes.

4. After 3 minutes, stop, sit down immediately, and take your pulse, counting every beat for 1 minute.

5. Consult Table 2.3 to determine your fitness category and to record your test results.[6]

6. Reassess your aerobic fitness progress at the conclusion of the course, recording these results on the post-test section of Table 2.3 and comparing your results. How did you change from the pre-test to post-test?

### Aerobic Fitness For Life

Before you begin your aerobic step training program, you should assess your cardiorespiratory endurance using one of the tests just presented, then reassess your cardiorespiratory efficiency 8 weeks later. As step training becomes a lifetime activity for you, you should be assessed every 2 months, and your results compared with those from your first assessment. This also will help you set continual, lifelong, specific physical fitness goals.

Attaining a level of physical fitness labeled "good" or "high" (lab tests), or "good," "excellent," or "superior" (field tests) does not mean you have achieved a finished product or goal. Instead, you have found a method of getting in shape that you must continue for the rest of your life.

The need for personal fitness must result in a complete change in lifestyle. You must prioritize and program exercise into your busy weekly schedule for the rest of your life. A yo-yo concept of a 10-week class now, and maybe one a year later, doesn't maintain fitness and a healthy heart.

### Goal Setting Aerobic Fitness

You have just completed assessing your *aerobic capacity*. With this information, you can establish your cardiovascular fitness goals. Setting goals helps to keep you focused on daily improvement and positive change. It encourages consistency in your fitness program and helps to keep you on target, because without goals there's nothing to shoot for.

Write one fitness goal to be achieved by the end of this course, on Tables 2.1, 2.2, or 2.3. Truly stretch yourself and your potential in regard to what you actually are capable of achieving.

At the conclusion of the course and after post-testing your progress, set a 2-month goal to work

toward. Life is a journey of small steps and successes. These require a process of continuous goal setting.

For some beginners, the "good" performance level is high. Do not be discouraged. You will be pleased with your improvement, as you participate in a regular step aerobics program.

### ■ Measuring Muscular Strength and Endurance

Although step training is basically a form of aerobic conditioning, it can also improve your muscular strength and endurance. Even though muscular strength and endurance are interrelated, they are different. *Strength* is the capacity of a muscle to exert maximal force against a resistance. *Endurance* is the capacity of a muscle to exert submaximal force repeatedly over a period of time. *Absolute strength* is usually determined by the maximal amount of resistance (one repetition maximum, or 1RM) that an individual can lift in a single effort. Because it requires access to a weight room and free weights or weight machines and some experience in weight training techniques, and it is not as easily tested in a step aerobics class, absolute strength will not be tested at this time.

Muscular endurance, on the other hand, is commonly determined by the number of reps (repetitions) an individual can perform against a submaximal resistance, or by the length of time that a given contraction can be sustained. Therefore, it can be tested easily and safely in the step aerobics setting. Determining your starting point will be beneficial in terms of your exercise progression. The following two tests give procedures for testing muscular endurance of your upper body and your abdomen.

### Push-Up Test

The push-up test can determine the muscular endurance of your *upper body*.

1. Lie face down on a mat or padded floor, and place your hands palm down under your shoulders. For males, begin in the standard push-up position with your body straight (Figure 2.2). Females may perform the modified push-up, in which the knees remain on the floor and the upper body and torso remain straight (do not bend at the hips) (Figure 2.3).

**TABLE 2.3 3-Minute Step Test: One Minute Post Exercise**

| Fitness Category | | Age (years) 18–25 | 26–35 | 36–45 | 46–55 | 56–65 | 65+ |
|---|---|---|---|---|---|---|---|
| | | Beats Per Minute | | | | | |
| I. Very Poor | (men) | >128 | >128 | >130 | >132 | >129 | >130 |
| | (women) | >140 | >138 | >140 | >135 | >139 | >134 |
| II. Poor | (men) | 117-128 | 118-128 | 120-130 | 123-132 | 121-129 | 121-130 |
| | (women) | 127-140 | 127-138 | 129-140 | 127-135 | 129-139 | 129-134 |
| III. Below Avg. | (men) | 106-116 | 108-117 | 113-119 | 117-122 | 113-120 | 114-120 |
| | (women) | 118-126 | 120-126 | 119-128 | 121-126 | 119-128 | 123-128 |
| IV. Average | (men) | 100-105 | 100-107 | 104-112 | 106-116 | 104-112 | 104-113 |
| | (women) | 109-117 | 112-119 | 111-118 | 116-120 | 113-118 | 116-122 |
| V. Above Avg. | (men) | 90-99 | 90-99 | 97-103 | 98-105 | 98-103 | 97-103 |
| | (women) | 99-108 | 100-111 | 103-110 | 105-115 | 105-112 | 103-115 |
| VI. Good | (men) | 79-89 | 81-89 | 83-96 | 87-97 | 86-97 | 88-96 |
| | (women) | 85-98 | 88-99 | 90-102 | 94-104 | 95-104 | 90-102 |
| VII. Excellent | (men) | <79 | <81 | <83 | <87 | <86 | <88 |
| | (women) | <85 | <88 | <90 | <94 | <95 | <90 |

< Means less than; > more than.

Source: Adapted from *The Y's Way to Physical Fitness*, 3d edition, by L. A. Golding, C. R. Meyers, and W. E. Sinning (1986). Reprinted by permission of the YMCA of the USA, 101 N. Wacker Drive. Chicago, IL 60606.

## PRE-TEST:

Name: ________________________________ Date: ______________

1-Minute Post-Exercise Heart Rate: ____________ bpm

**Circle Fitness Category:** Very Poor / Poor / Below Average / Average / Above Average / Good / Excellent

**COURSE GOAL:** ________________________________

## POST-TEST:

Name: ________________________________ Date: ______________

1-Minute Post-Exercise Heart Rate: ____________ bpm

**Circle Fitness Category:** Very Poor / Poor / Below Average / Average / Above Average / Good / Excellent

**2-MONTH GOAL:** ________________________________

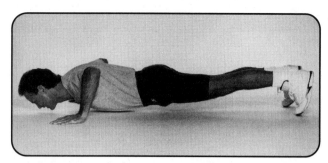

**Figure 2.2**  Standard Push-Up position.

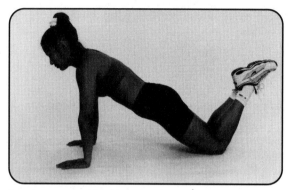

**Figure 2.3**  Modified Push-Up position.

2. Exhale as you extend your arms and lift your upper body and torso off the floor.

3. Lower your chest to within 3" of the floor.

4. Count the total number of non-stop push-ups you perform.

5. Refer to Table 2.4 to determine your fitness level.

6. Record your test results and set a course goal.

7. Reassess at the end of the course, record in the post-test section, and set a 2-month goal to work toward.

### Bent-Leg Sit-Up Test

The bent-leg sit-up test can determine the muscular strength and endurance of your *abdominal muscles.*

1. Lie on your back on a mat or padded floor and bend your knees so that your heels are 12"–18" from your buttocks.

2. Place your arms across your chest and have a partner hold your feet flat on the floor (Figure 2.4).

3. Contract your abdominals as you lift your shoulders and upper back upward and forward. At the top, at least one elbow must touch one knee (Figure 2.5).

4. Count one repetition each time you complete the cycle and return to the floor. Count the number of repetitions performed in 60 seconds.

5. Refer to Table 2.5 to determine your fitness level.

6. Record your test results and set a course goal.

7. Reassess at the end of the course, record in the post-test section, and set a 2-month goal to work toward.

### ▇▇ Measuring Flexibility

Flexibility is the ability of a specific joint and its corresponding muscle groups to move freely through its full range of motion. It is reflected in each individual's ability to bend and stretch at various specific joints. Because total range of motion about a joint is highly specific and the range varies greatly from one joint to the other and also from one person to another, it is rather difficult to precisely indicate how much flexibility is ideal overall.

Nevertheless, the participants in an aerobics class should have some indication of how flexible their lower back and hamstring (posterior, upper leg area) muscles are, as this area is significantly used in all aerobic activities. One exercise that tests the flexibility of this area is entitled the Modified Sit-and-Reach Test.

### Modified Sit-and-Reach Test

Some warm-up stretching of this area is advised before this test is administered.

1. Place a yardstick on top of a bench-step that is approximately 12" high (such as one Sports Step™ and four support blocks).

2. Remove your shoes and sit on the floor with your hips, back, and head against a wall and your legs fully extended, with the soles of your feet flat against the bench.

3. As shown in Figure 2.6, place your hands on top of each other, and reach forward as far as possible, *keeping your head and back against the wall.*

4. Instructor or partner slides the yardstick along the top of the bench until the end touches your fingertips (see arrow). The yardstick is now held firmly in place until your results are recorded.

5. Allow your back and head to come off the wall. Slowly stretch forward as far as possible along the top of the yardstick. Hold the position (see Figure 2.7) for several seconds, as the instructor

### TABLE 2.4　Push-Up Muscular Endurance Test Standards

Circle your gender and age.

| | Age (years) | Fitness Level | | | | | | |
| --- | --- | --- | --- | --- | --- | --- | --- | --- |
| | | Superior | Excellent | Very Good | Good | Average | Poor | Very Poor |
| **Males:** | | | | | | | | |
| **Push-Up** | 15-29 | 55+ | 51-54 | 45-50 | 35-44 | 25-34 | 20-24 | 15-19 |
| | 30-39 | 45+ | 41-44 | 35-40 | 25-34 | 20-24 | 15-19 | 8-14 |
| | 40-49 | 40+ | 35-39 | 30-34 | 20-29 | 14-19 | 12-13 | 5-11 |
| | 50-59 | 30+ | 26-29 | 20-25 | 10-19 | 8-9 | 5-7 | 0-4 |
| **Females:** | | | | | | | | |
| **Modified** | 15-29 | 49+ | 46-48 | 34-45 | 17-33 | 10-16 | 6-9 | 0-5 |
| **Push-Up** | 30-39 | 38+ | 34-37 | 25-33 | 12-24 | 8-11 | 4-7 | 0-3 |
| | 40-49 | 33+ | 29-32 | 20-28 | 8-19 | 6-7 | 3-5 | 0-2 |
| | 50-59 | 26+ | 22-25 | 15-21 | 6-14 | 4-5 | 2-3 | 0-1 |

Source: Adapted from *Fitness for College and Life*, 5th edition, 1997, by W. E. Prentice. Reprinted by permission of McGraw-Hill, 1221 Avenue of Americas, 45th Floor, New York, NY 10020.

## PRE-TEST:

Name: _____ Date: _____

Number of Push-Ups (non-stop and maintaining proper form): _____

**Circle Fitness Category:**　Very Poor / Poor / Average / Good / Very Good / Excellent / Superior

**COURSE GOAL:** _____

## POST-TEST:

Name: _____ Date: _____

Number of Push-Ups (non-stop and maintaining proper form): _____

**Circle Fitness Category:**　Very Poor / Poor / Average / Good / Very Good / Excellent / Superior

**2-MONTH GOAL:** _____

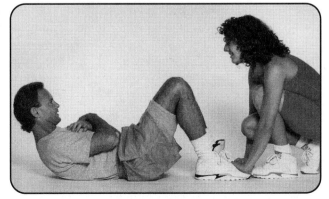

**Figure 2.4**　Starting position for Bent-Leg Sit-up.

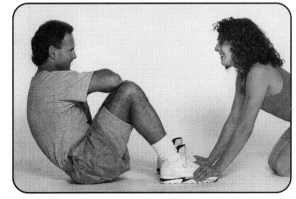

**Figure 2.5**　Up position for Bent-Leg Sit-up.

## TABLE 2.5    Bent-Knee Sit-Ups Test Standards

Circle your gender and age.

| | Age (years) | Superior | Excellent | Very Good | Good | Average | Poor | Very Poor |
|---|---|---|---|---|---|---|---|---|
| **Fitness Level** | | | | | | | | |
| **Males:** | 17-29 | 55+ | 51-55 | 48-50 | 42-47 | 36-41 | 17-35 | 0-17 |
| | 30-39 | 48+ | 44-48 | 39-43 | 33-38 | 27-32 | 13-26 | 0-13 |
| | 40-49 | 43+ | 39-43 | 34-38 | 28-33 | 23-27 | 11-22 | 0-11 |
| | 50-59 | 38+ | 34-38 | 29-33 | 22-28 | 17-21 | 8-16 | 0-8 |
| **Females:** | 17-29 | 47+ | 43-47 | 36-42 | 33-35 | 29-32 | 14-28 | 0-14 |
| | 30-39 | 45+ | 41-45 | 35-40 | 29-34 | 23-28 | 11-22 | 0-11 |
| | 40-49 | 40+ | 35-40 | 31-34 | 24-30 | 19-23 | 9-18 | 0-9 |
| | 50-59 | 35+ | 31-35 | 25-30 | 18-24 | 13-17 | 6-12 | 0-6 |

Source: *Fitness For College and Life,* 5th edition, 1997, by W. E. Prentice. Reprinted by permission of McGraw-Hill, 1221 Avenue of Americas, 45th Floor, New York, NY 10020.

## PRE-TEST:

Name: _____    Date: _____

Number of Sit-Ups Performed in 1 Minute: _____

**Circle Fitness Category:**   Very Poor / Poor / Average / Good / Very Good / Excellent / Superior

**COURSE GOAL:** _____

## POST-TEST:

Name: _____    Date: _____

Number of Sit-Ups Performed in 1 Minute: _____

**Circle Fitness Category:**   Very Poor / Poor / Average / Good / Very Good / Excellent / Superior

**2-MONTH GOAL:** _____

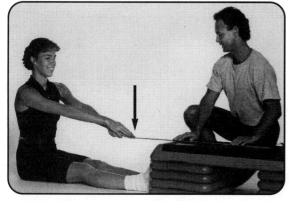

**Figure 2.6**   Determining the starting position for Modified Sit-and-Reach.

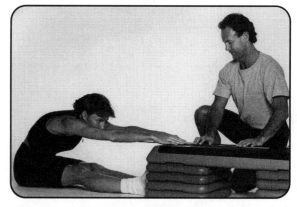

**Figure 2.7**   Modified Sit-and-Reach Test.

or partner determines, to the nearest ½", the exact total number of inches you reached. Mentally note results.

6. Repeat this procedure two more times. Use the average of the three trials as your Modified Sit-and-Reach Test score. Using Table 2.6, according to your age and gender, determine both your percentile rank and flexibility classification for this test,[7] recording your results and setting a course goal.

7. Reassess at the end of the course, record in the post-test section, and set a 2-month goal to work toward.

Unlike the traditional Sit-and-Reach Test, the *modified* protocol used here varies in that the arm and leg lengths are taken into consideration to determine your score. (In the original test procedures, the 15" mark of the yardstick is always set at the edge of the box where the feet are placed.

**TABLE 2.6 Percentile Ranks and Total Inches Measured for Modified Sit-And-Reach Test**

Circle your gender and age categories.

**Flexibility**

| **Men** | **Age Category** | | | | **Women** | **Age Category** | | | |
|---|---|---|---|---|---|---|---|---|---|
| **Percentile Rank** | **<18** | **19–35** | **36–49** | **50>** | **Percentile Rank** | **<18** | **19–35** | **36–49** | **50>** |
| 99 | 20.8 | 20.1 | 18.9 | 16.2 | 99 | 22.6 | 21.0 | 19.8 | 17.2 |
| 95 | 19.6 | 18.9 | 18.2 | 15.8 | 95 | 19.5 | 19.3 | 19.2 | 15.7 |
| 90 | 18.2 | 17.2 | 16.1 | 15.0 | 90 | 18.7 | 17.9 | 17.4 | 15.0 |
| 80 | 17.8 | 17.0 | 14.6 | 13.3 | 80 | 17.8 | 16.7 | 16.2 | 14.2 |
| 70 | 16.0 | 15.8 | 13.9 | 12.3 | 70 | 16.5 | 16.2 | 15.2 | 13.6 |
| 60 | 15.2 | 15.0 | 13.4 | 11.5 | 60 | 16.0 | 15.8 | 14.5 | 12.3 |
| 50 | 14.5 | 14.4 | 12.6 | 10.2 | 50 | 15.2 | 14.8 | 13.5 | 11.1 |
| 40 | 14.0 | 13.5 | 11.6 | 9.7 | 40 | 14.5 | 14.5 | 12.8 | 10.1 |
| 30 | 13.4 | 13.0 | 10.8 | 9.3 | 30 | 13.7 | 13.7 | 12.2 | 9.2 |
| 20 | 11.8 | 11.6 | 9.9 | 8.8 | 20 | 12.6 | 12.6 | 11.0 | 8.3 |
| 10 | 9.5 | 9.2 | 8.3 | 7.8 | 10 | 11.4 | 10.1 | 9.7 | 7.5 |
| 05 | 8.4 | 7.9 | 7.0 | 7.2 | 05 | 9.4 | 8.1 | 8.5 | 3.7 |
| 01 | 7.2 | 7.0 | 5.1 | 4.0 | 01 | 6.5 | 2.6 | 2.0 | 1.5 |

| **Fitness Categories** | |
|---|---|
| **Percentile Rank** | **Fitness Category** |
| 81> | Excellent |
| 61–80 | Good |
| 41–60 | Average |
| 21–40 | Fair |
| <20 | Poor |

High physical fitness standard

Health fitness standard

Source: *Principles & Labs for Physical Fitness and Wellness,* by Werner W. K. Hoeger (Englewood, CO: Morton Publishing, 1991), p. 135.

**PRE-TEST:**

Name: ______________________________ Date: ______________

Total Inches Measured: ______________________________

**Circle Fitness Category:** Poor / Fair / Average / Good / Excellent **COURSE GOAL:** ______________

**POST-TEST:**

Name: ______________________________ Date: ______________

Total Inches Measured: ______________________________

**Circle Fitness Category:** Poor / Fair / Average / Good / Excellent **2-MONTH GOAL:** ______________

This procedure does not differentiate between an individual with long arms and short legs and someone with short arms and long legs. All other factors being equal, the individual with the longer arms and shorter legs would receive a better rating because of the structural advantage.[8]

## SUMMARY

Fitness testing pre-assessments are a great way to determine your fitness level or category in the physical fitness components of cardiovascular endurance, muscular strength and endurance and flexibility. The results will give you an indication of your physical readiness to start a step training program or to determine if you should progress to a more demanding training program. You may find that you are fit in one component but need to improve in another area.

Take the tests before you begin (or continue) your training program to determine your starting points, and retake the tests after 8 to 12 weeks to monitor your progress. It is exciting to actually see positive results from your efforts and it will help to motivate you to adhere to your program.

If you don't see immediate improvements, don't be discouraged. You may need to modify your training to get the results you want. Your personal exercise plan should be one that helps you to improve your physical weaknesses, while at the same time improving your physical strengths.

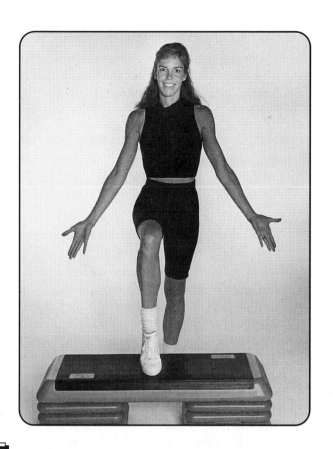

# THE NEXT STEP: BECOMING AN INFORMED STEPPER

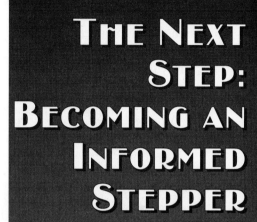

The next step ...........................ld becoming efficient at ....................... provides many challen.......................needs. Bench/step training ...........................train-ing continues to be ...........................ining, much research has ...........................iologi-cal and biomechan...........................ollow-ing information ar.............................various researchers promc...........................noting products to use wit

## ■ Benefits

Step training invo...........................rm or bench, adding a ....................................further challenge. It is kn...........................or step aerobics, bench o..........................ping.

The key advantage to a step training program over other aero-bics is that it is primarily a high-intensity activity used to pro-mote cardiovascular and respiratory fitness but with low impact to satisfy safety concerns. A vast majority of all the moves in-volves one foot supporting the weight, either on the bench plat-form or on the floor. Other benefits include the following:

▌ It's a terrific conditioning workout for every major muscle group in the lower body, specifically the hamstrings, quadriceps, gluteals, and calves.

▌ Upper torso movements provide conditioning work for muscles of the arms, shoulders, chest, and back, and therefore a balanced and complete workout that strengthens and tones the entire body. This becomes especially apparent later if you combine training modes within one class format (see Chapter 7) or perform step and strength intervals (see Chapter 8).

■ The basic moves are simple. By introducing various step patterns with fewer (or more) arm gestures, adjusting the height of the bench, increasing or decreasing the range of motion used, incorporating long or short levers and incorporating propulsion or low impact moves, participants of all ages, skill and fitness levels, and both genders can be challenged simultaneously.

> *An effective cardiovascular workout has aerobic benefits equal to running 7 miles per hour (mph), yet has the potentially low-impact equivalence of walking at a 3 mph pace, minimizing the chance of injury.*[6]

## ■ Research Findings

Step training is similar to all other forms of physical activity because it has an element of risk. The concerns and subsequent research associated with this new modality of exercise have focused on evaluating:

1. Energy cost of aerobic bench/step techniques
2. Physiological benefits
3. Musculoskeletal safety of step training exercise.[7,8,9,10,11,12]

Research to date has produced the following highlights:

■ Step training provides the sufficient cardiovascular and respiratory demands needed to attain cardiovascular and respiratory fitness in accordance with American College of Sports Medicine (ACSM) guidelines.[13]

■ Determining exact energy costs depends upon various factors including height of the step bench, rate of stepping, and step pattern/technique.[14]

■ Bench step height and rate of stepping significantly affect metabolic cost. This varies among participants because of differences in muscle mass rather than height of participants.[15]

■ Specific step moves used within a workout all have specific effects on energy cost (that is, different movement patterns result in different intensities perceived or achieved). For example, moves such as the basic step, step touch, and bypass moves expend less energy than lunging, traveling, and repeater moves.[16]

■ Propulsion or power movements significantly increase heart rate and exercise intensity.[17]

■ Stepping at accelerated speeds (33–35 cycles per minute) result in an increase in lactic acid levels indicating anaerobic metabolism.[18]

■ Step training injuries vary with the ground force impact and are related to step height, speed of music, and movements performed.[19]

In summary, and in keeping with current research data, step training performed according to ACSM guidelines can significantly improve cardiovascular fitness. And because several variables can affect heart rate intensity, programs can be designed to meet the needs of each individual participant, to facilitate both optimum safety and effectiveness.

## ■ Choosing Your Bench Height

When choosing a bench height, each of the following factors should be considered.

■ Beginners who have not exercised regularly, have limited coordination, or have no experience in step training should select a 4" to 6" bench initially. (For the 12" bench pictured, this represents the basic 4" platform and, at most, one 2" support block on each end.)

■ Intermediate or regular step trainers with a "physically fit" level of cardiovascular and respiratory fitness should choose an 8" to 10" bench. (An 8" bench equals the platform plus two 2" support blocks; or, for a 10" bench, three 2" support blocks).

■ Advanced, or skilled regular step trainers with a high level of cardiovascular fitness should choose a 10" to 12" bench (the platform plus a maximum of four support blocks on each end).

■ Taller people and those with longer legs than most people should consider using a bench of 8" to 12".

■ Regardless of level of fitness or experience, the bench height should not allow the knee to flex less than 90 degrees (Figure 3.1) when the knee is weight-bearing. If the knees advance *beyond the toes* while stepping up, the platform is too high.

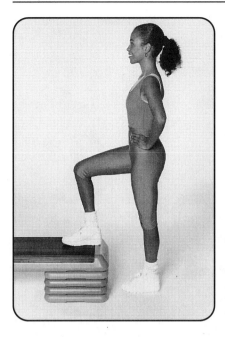

**Figure 3.1** If the knees advance beyond your toes as you step up, the platform is too high.

Choosing a platform that is too high for your energy or fitness level may affect your body alignment and result in injury. For example, if you are leaning too far forward, the platform may be too high and can cause undesirable pressure on the lower back.[20]

An optional test for bench height is shown in Figure 3.2: Place one foot flat on top of the bench; allow a 3" drop from the hip to knee for safe movement up to the top of the bench.

## ■ Music

As the underlying structure of a step training program, music plays a significant role. Fun, exciting music can motivate and challenge participants. The tempo of the music (measured as beats per minute) directs the progression of movement and also the speed of the movements. Movements have to be controlled, and music with a bpm (beats per minute) of 118 to 125 is best,[21] so be sure to select music with the appropriate tempo (Figure 3.3).

Stepping at speeds above the recommended guidelines can be unsafe and can result in the following: [22]

■ Poor postural alignment because of the tendency to bend forward at the waist in order to step onto the platform more quickly.

■ Improper foot placement and inability to make full foot contact with the bench when stepping up, and the floor when stepping back.

■ Limited range of motion, particularly for long-limbed individuals.

■ Increase in ground force impact, which has the potential to cause overuse injuries.

The music should have a clear beat that is easy to follow. Following are the suggested tempos to use for the segment durations.[23]

| Duration (minutes) | Segment | bpm |
| --- | --- | --- |
| 10–12 | Warm-Up | 130–140 |
| 4–5 | Pre-Aerobic | 118–124 |
| 20–30 | Aerobic Stepping | 122–126 |
| 4–5 | Post-Aerobic | 120–124 |
| 10–15 | Muscle Conditioning | 110–130 |
| 5–6 | Slow Stretch | <100 |

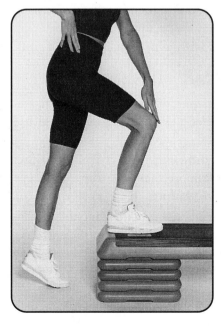

**Figure 3.2** Allow a 3" drop from the hip to knee.

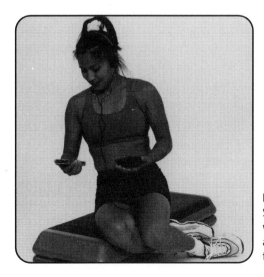

**Figure 3.3.** Select music with the appropriate tempo.

## ■ Body Alignment and Stepping Technique

Good posture is required for a safe, injury-free workout. Proper alignment and stepping technique include the following:

■ Keep your back straight, head and chest up, shoulders back, abdomen tight, and buttocks tucked under hips, with eyes on the platform (Figure 3.4).

■ As much as possible, keep your shoulders aligned over your hips. Lean forward with the whole body. Don't bend from the hips or round the shoulders and lean forward or backward.

■ Step up lightly to avoid unnecessary high impact, and make sure the whole foot lands on the platform, with the heel bearing your weight. Partial foot placement on the bench (with the heel off the bench) increases your chance of slipping off the bench, tripping, or even flipping the bench.

■ Keep your knees aligned over your feet when they're pulling your body weight onto the platform.

■ At the top, straighten your legs but don't lock your knees. Keep them "soft."

■ As you step down, stay close to the platform. Step down, not back. Land on the ball of the foot (Figure 3.4), then bring the heel down onto the floor before taking the next step. Stepping too far back with the leading leg causes the body to lean slightly forward, placing extra stress on the foot, achilles, and calf.

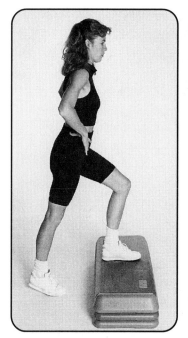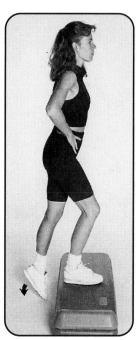

**Figure 3.4** Proper technique for stepping up and stepping down.

## Stepping[24]

■ Avoid excessive arm movements over your head, as this places a great deal of stress on the shoulder joint.

■ Maintain appropriate speed for safe and effective movement.

■ Change the lead leg after 1 minute maximum. The lead leg (leg that steps up first) experiences the most muscular skeletal stress.

■ Limit propulsions and power moves. Power movements are considered advanced and can result in greater ground force impact. Power or propulsion steps should be performed only **onto** the step and not down.

■ Do not perform more than 8 counts (4 repeaters) on one leg at a time, as repeated foot impact without variation is potentially harmful.

■ Do not pivot or twist the knee on the weight-bearing leg.

■ Do not step up with your back toward the platform.

■ Limit propulsions and power moves.

■ Maintain muscular balance, working opposing muscle groups equally (quadriceps/hamstrings; calves/tibialis anterior; pectorals/upper back).

■ If you feel faint or dizzy or if any exercise causes pain or severe discomfort, stop the exercise immediately but continue to move around.

■ Do not allow anyone to perform on the bench with you. Only one person at a time should use the bench.

■ For the bench shown in the chapter opening photo, do not use more than four support blocks on each end of the platform.

■ If you are pregnant, check with your doctor before starting this program. If you are cleared by your doctor, make certain that you keep your heart rate at 23 beats or below for a 10-second count (138 bpm). A step height of no more than 6" is recommended during pregnancy.

# CORRECT STEP TRAINING POSTURE

Three common step training errors and their corrections are illustrated in Figures 3.5–3.10. The man is demonstrating incorrect postural techniques for each exercise, and the woman is performing correctly. Additional performance suggestions are also included.[25]

**These moves are important to include for muscle balance:**

**Figure 3.5
Errors in hip/leg extension**
Some participants create an undesirable curve of the lower back with an excessive rear leg lift and exaggerate the problem with a forward body lean.

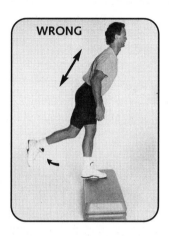

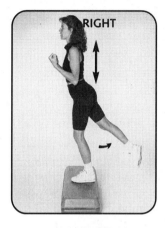

**Figure 3.6
Correction for hip-leg extension**
Stand tall on the platform and extend the rear lifting leg **back**, not up.

**These moves are great exercises for the thighs and buttocks:**

**Figure 3.7
Errors in side step-out squats**
Some participants have a tendency to lean too far out to the side, which places too much stress on the knee.

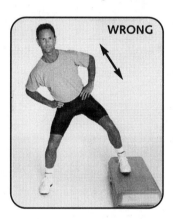

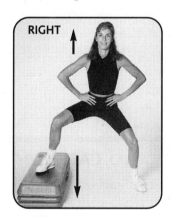

**Figure 3.8
Correction for side step-out squats**
Balance your weight evenly, keeping your center of gravity squarely within your legs.

**Figure 3.9
Errors in step-back lunges from platform**
Some participants bend too far forward at the hip or have the leg reaching back in a locked-knee position. Also, the heel should not be forced to the ground; this position may be too much dorsiflexion of the foot for you.

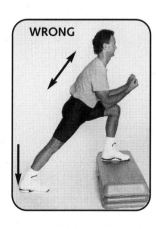

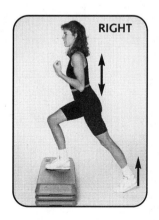

**Figure 3.10   Correction for step-back lunges from platform**   Keep your body weight predominantly over the platform leg, and keep your knee over your toes. The leg reaching back should make floor contact, with your knee slightly flexed. This will help reduce any chance of joint trauma from ground impact. The back heel is raised off the floor.

## Lifting and Lowering

▌ Use correct lifting and lowering techniques. To protect your muscles and joints (especially the lower back) from undue strain or fatigue, proper, efficient technique in these areas must become second nature to you. Disciplined practice of correct techniques now will establish good habits for the rest of your life. The leg muscles are very strong, whereas the back muscles are relatively weak. All heavy lifting should be done by stabilizing the back in an erect position and making the *legs* provide the necessary power.

▌ Get as close to the object as possible, using a forward-stride position. The object should be in front of you if you are using two hands (as in the step bench) or beside you if you are using one hand (such as luggage). Keep your back straight and your pelvis tucked, and bend at the hips, knees, and ankles to lower your body. Lower directly downward, only as much as necessary.

▌ Place both arms well under or *around the weight center* of the load. Lift vertically upward in a slow, steady movement by extending your leg muscles. Keep the object close to your weight center (see Figure 3.11). Reverse the procedure to lower the object.

▌ *Do not* bend over from the hips (head low, buttocks high), as that would make your back muscles lift the load (see Figure 3.12).

## Correct Carrying

▌ Keep the object close to your weight center.

▌ Separate the load when feasible, and carry half in each hand/arm (see Figure 3.13).

## ▬ Shoe Selection

The shoes you wear constitute one of your major requirements. When you jump or run, you place three to six times more force on your feet than when you are not using them. If you weigh 125 pounds, you are placing 375 to 750 pounds of pressure on your feet with each jump. Your body can withstand the stress of exercise better if you wear shoes that shock-absorb this pressure or exercise on a surface with a "giving" quality.

Because step training puts a great deal of stress on the achilles tendon and calf, the shoe should have sufficient heel lift to absorb this impact. The shoe also should bend easily behind the toes, because when stepping down from the platform, you land on the ball of the foot and then bring the heel down.

The following criteria[26] give specific guidelines for personalizing your shoe selection.

▌ Inquire about midsole composition. For durability and performance, select shoes made from either compression-molded ethyl vinyl acetate (EVA) or polyurethane.

## CORRECT LIFTING AND CARRYING

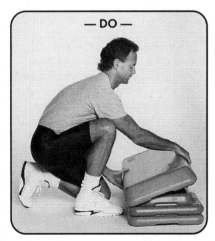

**Figure 3.11**  Correct lifting technique.

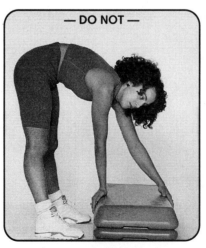

**Figure 3.12**  Incorrect lifting technique.

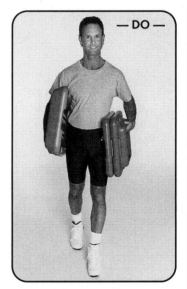

**Figure 3.13**  Correct carrying technique.

- Stay with the same brand and model of shoe you are replacing if it has been satisfactory.

- Do not allow yourself to be forced or pressured into buying a shoe that does not feel comfortable.

- About every 4 months replace a single pair of shoes worn at least 4 days per week for any fitness-related activity. If the shoes have a polyurethane midsole, the wear may be extended up to 6 months. If they have a standard, open-cell EVA midsole, they may last only 3 months.

- Examine the inside of the shoe as well as the insole. Shoes with removable insoles are preferable because they tend to be better cushioned and allow the fit of a custom foot orthotic, if needed.[27]

- Get nylon uppers rather than leather uppers if you want a cooler shoe. If you prefer an all-leather shoe, be sure it has ventilation holes on the top and sides. Extra design leather or suede along the ball edge of the foot area (toes) provides longer shoe life.

- Choose a shoe that has a sole with a relatively smooth tread[28] and of white rubber, designed for aerobics or court use (Figure 3.14).

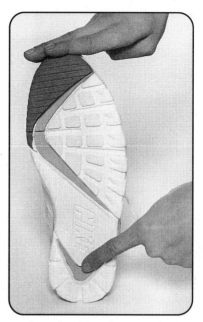

**Figure 3.14**　Sole with rubber designed for sideward movement, and heel unflared.

The rough treads of most running shoes can be hazardous during aerobic exercise dance accompanying your step training program, as they can cause the feet to come to an abrupt halt each time they strike the floor. Thus, most shoes designed for running are unsuitable for the aerobic dance intervals.[29]

Select a shoe that feels comfortable to you. Improper fitting or poorly designed shoes can be uncomfortable and lead to injury. The purpose of footwear is to support the foot, protect the foot and improve traction. The right choice will make your experience more enjoyable.

## SUMMARY

A bench/step training program has many advantages and benefits. It is a high-intensity exercise that sustains the training zone heart-rate needed to produce the cardiovascular and respiratory training effect. Yet, it is low-impact and safe, as one foot remains on the bench or the ground. Maintaining the safety precautions of selecting the correct bench height, good body positioning and alignment, and variety in technique, to prevent over-use, all work together to establish an exciting modality of aerobics training.

At this point you have an understanding of the most important step: *personal safety*. It is now time to begin your step training program, and this is initiated by making a written/verbal commitment to yourself regarding working on your personal fitness this term. Take a moment and fill out Exercise 3.1 entitled, "A Commitment To Fitness." This activity greatly assists in establishing the mental aspect of your training program, because it provides for the acknowledgment of your pre-tested starting points, and encourages the idea of pre-course goal-setting.

**EXERCISE 3.1**

## A COMMITMENT TO FITNESS

I, _____ (name),

am determined that today _____ (date),
am committed to becoming fit!

I acknowledge that I am in need of improvement in various facets of my well-being (physical, social, emotional, spiritual, intellectual, talent expression) and commit to devote _____ minutes **EVERY** day toward making positive change in my fitness habits. This is in addition to the time I spend in class.

The best time of day for me to work on this change is _____. At this very moment, I am scheduling it on my date book, just for me.

Absolutely **NOTHING** will take precedence over this block of time that I have set aside for personal fitness gains.

The short-term goals I am immediately taking direct action on include the following. (Be sure to mark only those you are choosing to change/improve):

▌ Cardiovascular (aerobic)
days per week sessions
(for at least 20 mins.)                    From: _____     To: _____

▌ Flexibility sit and reach test results   From: –/+ _____"   To: –/+ _____"

▌ Muscular strength and endurance
of abdominals (sit-ups per workout)        From: _____     To: _____

▌ Muscular strength and endurance
of upper body (pushups per workout)        From: _____     To: _____

▌ Other goals (i.e., specific new, better choices)

_____          From: _____     To: _____

_____          From: _____     To: _____

                                           Today's                Completion
Signed _____     Date: _____       Date: _____

This commitment was witnessed by* _____ Date _____

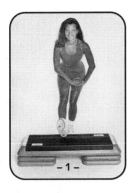

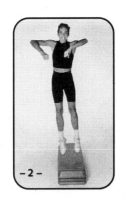

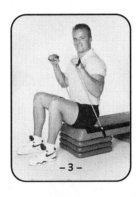

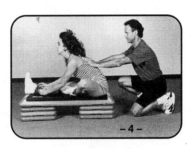

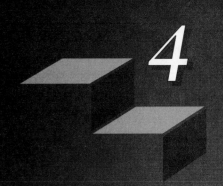

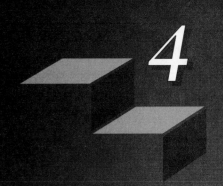
n effective step training fitness workout encompasses the following segments: (1) warm-up/stretch, (2) step aerobics, (3) strength training/muscle conditioning exercises, and (4) cool-down, flexibility, and relaxation. When these segments are incorporated into your step training program, you can achieve overall physical fitness. Using the following principles and guidelines for each segment will help to achieve the results you desire.[1, 2, 3, 4, 5]

## Warm-Up Segment

The warm-up begins with active, low-level, rhythmic, limbering, standing, range-of-motion types of exercises that raise the body's core temperature slightly, initiate muscular movements, and prepare you for more strenuous moves to come. Moves on the step-bench integrate use of both the floor and the bench. An example is to perform bench step taps with bicep curls (Figure 4.1).

Use low-impact moves that allow you to adjust to the height and contour of the bench, such as stepping up and down at half the tempo, marching on top of the bench, or straddling the bench and alternating tapping on top of the bench (Figure 4.2). The time-frame for the warm-up is approximately 5 minutes.

After the muscles, tendons, ligaments, and joints are loose and pliable, exercise takes the form of slow, sustained, static stretching. Static stretching — probably the most popular,

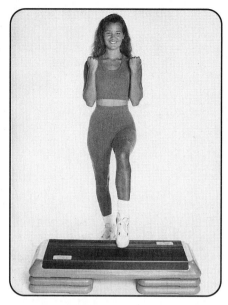

**Figure 4.1** Bench step taps, with bicep curls.

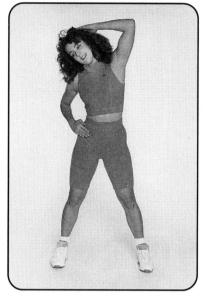

**Figure 4.3** Drop head to the side and press.

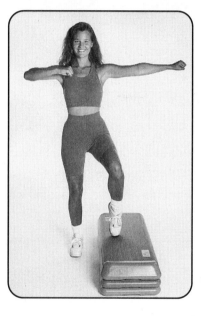

**Figure 4.2** Alternate tapping on top, from the straddle position.

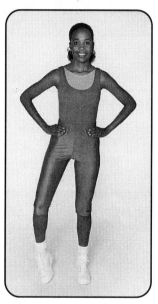 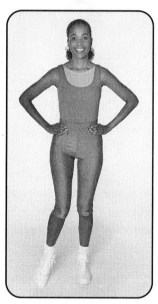

**Figure 4.4** Ankle stretching, circling out and circling in.

easiest, and safest form of stretching — involves gradually stretching a muscle or muscle group to the point of limitation, then holding that position for approximately 15 seconds. The stretch is repeated to the opposite side. Several repetitions of each stretch are performed. Static stretching is recommended when muscles are *warm* (after the initial active phase of the warm-up and later after intense physical activity).

Stretch all major muscles from head to toe (Figures 4.3 and 4.4), with special consideration for the major muscle groups in the legs, such as the thighs, hips, and calves, as step training is lower-body

intensive. When step training, the bench can be used as a fixed object to enhance stretching (Figures 4.5–4.10).[6]

Breathe continuously. Your entire system, especially your working muscles, constantly need oxygen. Holding your breath and turning red is never an appropriate way to exercise. When you stretch, exhale by puckering your lips and breathing out, and inhale when you relax your muscles.

Cue yourself: "Breathe out and stretch. Breathe in and relax."

The timeframe for the warm-up stretching segment is approximately 5 minutes.

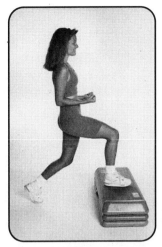

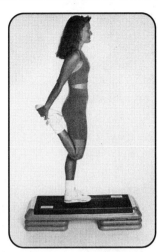

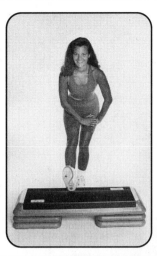

**Figure 4.5** Hip flexors — facing the bench.

**Figure 4.6** Quadricep stretch — standing on the bench.

**Figure 4.7** Hamstring stretch — facing the bench.

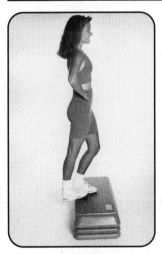

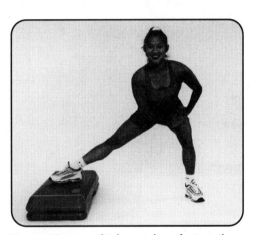

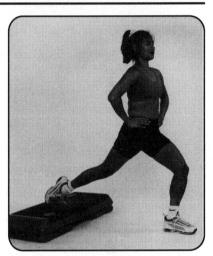

**Figure 4.8** Calf stretch — standing on top of the bench.

**Figure 4.9** Inner thigh stretch — foot on the bench.

**Figure 4.10** Anterior tibialis (front of lower leg) — top of foot on the bench.

## ▣ Step Aerobics Segment

The aerobics segment can be subdivided into sections, each focusing on its impact in relation to the heart rate intensity you are building, sustaining, or lowering, and according to the phase of the session you're in. You should monitor your heart rate at least twice during the 30–40 minute segment.

This segment begins with the *pre-aerobic* phase, a progressive transition from the warm-up into the high-intensity aerobic phase. As an example, perform basic steps with a variety of arm movements as shown in Figure 4.11. Pre-aerobic moves are performed at a moderate tempo to gradually increase the body's temperature and heart rate.

During the aerobic segment, the intensity of the exercises (measured as heart rate bpm) should in-crease gradually to your fitness level. Vary your movements to maintain your interest, ensure safety, and effectively work as many muscles as possible. Begin by coordinating the arms and the legs (Figure 4.12), then build more difficult movement patterns (Figures 4.13 and 4.14).

Finally, to provide a transition between the vigorous aerobic work and the anaerobic strength training segment of the workout, the heart rate must be gradually brought back down to the normal (pre-exercise) heart rate. This helps prevent a build-up of lactic acid (metabolic waste product) and keeps the blood from pooling in the lower extremities.

Like the pre-aerobic phase, the *post-aerobic cool-down* is performed at a slower tempo. It consists of lower range-of-motion movements such as those illustrated in Figures 4.15 and 4.16.

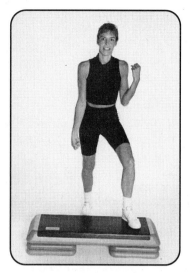

**Figure 4.11** V-step with bicep curl.

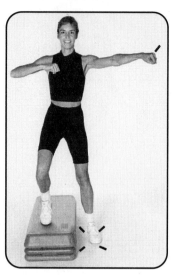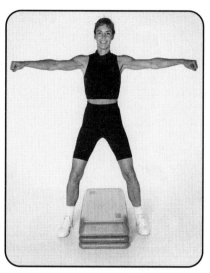

**Figure 4.12** Straddle down using coordinated arm movements.

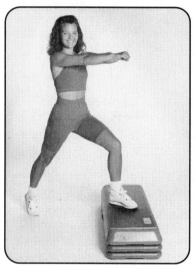

**Figures 4.13**
Lunge right.
Continue by
building more
difficult movement
patterns.

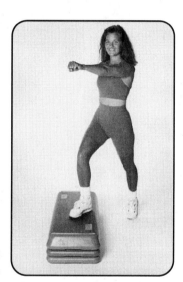

**Figures 4.14**
Lunge left.

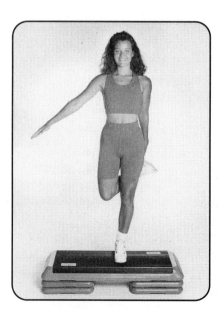

**Figure 4.15** Post-
aerobic cool down:
Hamstring curl
touch heel in back.

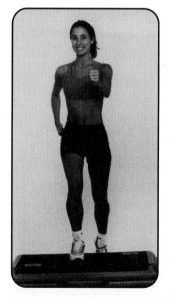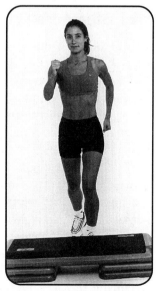

**Figure 4.16** Post-aerobic cool-down — mambo: step forward
and step back.

# Muscle Conditioning/ Strength Training Segment

During vigorous aerobics, all muscles of the body are strengthened. The strength segment included within an aerobics workout, focusing on the strength development of isolated muscle groups, follows the aerobics workout and comes before the final cool-down, flexibility training, and relaxation segments.

The reasoning is simple. With an increase in the resistance (weight) that must be applied to any movement for significant change (training) to occur, the workload placed on the heart, lungs, and vascular system also increases. An individual is more readily placed in a breathless "oxygen-debt" state. During the aerobic phase, the goal is *not* to be in a breathless state but, instead, in a breathe-easy state, steadily pacing the intensity.

The muscle conditioning/strength training segment focuses on specific muscle groups in a steady, controlled manner (which tends to sustain proper body postural alignment), *concentrating on areas not adequately worked during the aerobic segment.* In contrast to step aerobics, which is lower-body-intensive, this segment works the muscles in the upper body and the abdominals, in two or three sets of 8 to 12 repetitions. This prescription is for all muscle groups except for the abdominals. Repetitions can be increased to 15–30 for each of the two sets for the abdominals.

To incorporate variety into the strength training segment, different forms of resistance, such as hand-held weights, resistance bands, and tubing, can be used. Sample strength/bench exercises that work isolated muscle groups are: for the chest, push-ups (Figure 4.17) and bent-arm chest cross-over (Figure 4.18); for the arms and shoulders, short-lever bicep curls (Figure 4.19) and long-lever lateral raises (Figure 4.20); for the abdomen,

curl-up variations (Figure 4.21); and for the buttocks, squats (Figure 4.22).

These exercises are done to more quickly define, tone, shape, and make more dense (thicken) the muscle fibers. They also allow longer periods of work during the exercise program and later in daily work tasks. Chapter 8 provides principles, guidelines, and suggested exercises for safe, effective strength training.

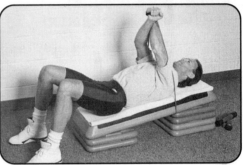

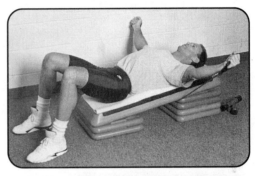

**Figure 4.18** Bent-Arm Chest Cross-Over (tubing) — for the chest.

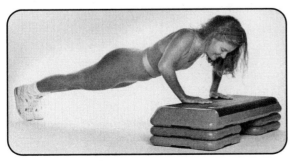

**Figure 4.17** Push-up on the bench (your weight) — for the chest.

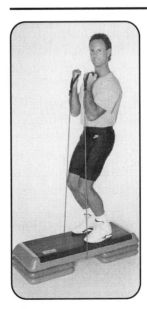

**Figure 4.19** Short-lever bicep curls (tubing) — for arms and shoulders.

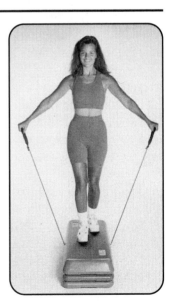

**Figure 4.20** Long-lever lateral raises (tubing) — for arms and shoulders.

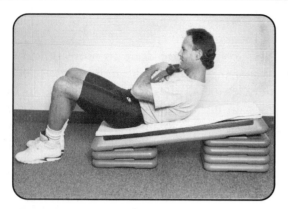

**Figure 4.21** Gravity-assisted Curl-Up (incline bench and 1-4 lb. weights) — for abdominals.

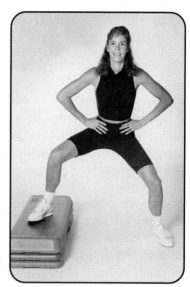

**Figure 4.22** Squats (bench) — for buttocks.

## ■ Cool-Down, Flexibility, and Relaxation Segment

The purpose of a cool-down segment in the workout is to give the body time to readjust to the pre-activity state. This eases the gradual process of returning the large quantity of blood now in the working muscles (primarily in the arms and legs) toward the vital organs in the head and trunk. Abruptly stopping a highly strenuous activity session may cause the blood to "pool" or stay in the extremities (primarily in the legs, because the veins of the legs are not being forcefully squeezed now by strenuously working the leg muscles). This pooling can cause cramping, nausea, dizziness, and fainting, as the needed quantity of oxygen and blood is not being delivered to the brain and other vital organs.

The ability to recover from exertion usually determines the duration of cool-down. A minimum of 5 to 10 minutes is essential, however, (a) to curtail profuse sweating, and (b) to lower the heart rate to below 120 beats per minute. These are two visible signs to monitor and achieve before concluding the exercise hour.

You'll begin the cooling down process by slowing down all large-muscle activity. Tapering off the activity level can be done in various ways, such as performing slow-tempo, low-impact step aerobics moves (Figure 4.23). This segment begins the transition between the vigorous bench/strength activity, just completed, and the flexibility training and relaxation performed last.

## Flexibility Training

Flexibility refers to the *range-of-motion of a given joint and its corresponding muscle groups*. It is genetically influenced and highly specific varying from joint to joint within an individual. When repeatedly stretched, muscle can be lengthened by approximately 20 percent.[7] In contrast, tendons can increase in length only about 2%–3%.

Flexibility training, or *stretching*, is widely accepted as an effective means of increasing joint mobility, improving exercise performance, and reducing injuries.[8] Proper technique is essential, for the risks of injury may be significant if stretches are performed incorrectly.

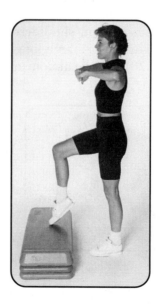

**Figure 4.23** Cool-down with a step tap.

Stretching programs follow the principle of **specific adaptation to imposed demands (SAID)**, which states that an individual must slowly and progressively stretch the soft tissues around a joint to and slightly beyond the point of limitation but not to the point of tearing.

At present, the two most widely accepted methods of stretching for improving flexibility are static and proprioceptive neuromuscular facilitatory (PNF) techniques. Both techniques follow the philosophy that flexibility is increased and risk of injury is prevented when the muscle being stretched is as relaxed as possible.

## STATIC STRETCHING

*Static stretching* is slow, active stretching, and the position is held at the joint extremes. The technique for executing stretching efficiently and safely is to gently ease into a controlled, stretched position and hold it as you gently press (Figure 4.24). Push or press to the point of tightness, "stretch pull" (a tight feeling but not a pain) so you feel the muscle working.

Continue to stretch a little beyond this point without any motion. Mentally relax and hold the position for approximately 15 seconds, allowing the muscle to also relax and feel heavier.[9] Continue to relax, and slowly withdraw the stretch. The same stretching on the opposite side of the body follows.

At present, static stretching is considered to be one of the most effective methods of increasing flexibility. Research has shown that significant gains can be achieved with a training program of static stretching exercises. This type of continuous, long stretching produces greater flexibility with less possibility of injury, probably because it stretches the muscles under controlled conditions.

## PNF STRETCHING

*PNF stretching*, in which muscles are stretched progressively with intermittent isometric contractions, is also effective in increasing flexibility and is used, like static stretches, when the muscles are warm. Two of the most commonly used modified PNF stretches are:

1. *Contract-relax technique:* In phase one, the exerciser does a 5- to 6-second maximum voluntary contraction in the muscle to be stretched. The contraction is isometric because any motion is resisted. In phase two, the previously contracted muscle is relaxed, then stretched.

2. *Agonist contract-relax technique:* In phase one, the exerciser maximally contracts the muscle opposite the muscle to be stretched against resistance (a partner, the floor, or other immovable object) for 5 to 6 seconds. In phase two, the agonist muscle is relaxed and the antagonist muscle is stretched.[10]

An example of a forward PNF contract-relax exercise for the hamstrings and spinal extensors, shown in Figure 4.25, is performed with a partner's assistance. The position and actions are detailed.

▪ *Position:* In a modified hurdler stretch position, the performing partner leans forward to the point of limitation while keeping the back straight and the toes of the extended leg facing upward to correctly stretch the hamstrings.

▪ *Action:* To begin the action, the performer pushes the back against the partner (contracting the spinal extensors) and pushes the extended leg against the floor (contracting the hamstrings) for a 6-second isometric contraction. The partner gently but firmly resists any movement.

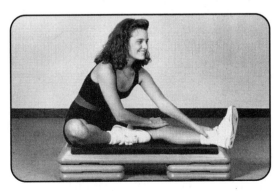

**Figure 4.24** Static stretching.

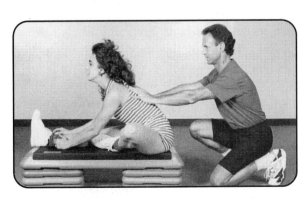

**Figure 4.25** PNF stretching

■ *Action*: After releasing the contraction, the performer stretches to a new point of limitation, holding a static stretch for 12 seconds or more while the partner maintains a light pressure on the performer's back.

Research has shown that *both* static and PNF techniques for stretching are effective. Each can be used successfully to enhance flexibility.

## Time to Stretch

Stretching to increase flexibility and range of motion is crucial now. It is a time when the muscles are warm (full of blood, oxygen, and nutrients) and the joints are pliable from vigorous exercise. Take full advantage of the next 5 to 10 minutes to static or PNF stretch (Figures 4.26–4.29).

## Static Stretching with Relaxation

Relaxation techniques complete the total physical fitness session and can begin during the stretching phase (Figure 4.30), to realize greater flexibility gains, and continue when stretching is completed, when muscle tension is absent throughout the body (Figure 4.31).

The participant focuses on three key factors:

1. Mental images
2. Self-talk accompanying each stretch and release (or PNF contract-relax and stretch, according to which technique you are using)
3. Mechanics of your breathing pattern.

The mental images now match the accompanying self-talk. The muscles being isolated and stretched are pictured and affirmed as becoming "wider, and longer, warmer and heavier."

Your breathing pattern is sequenced with these pictures and affirmations. An 8-count deep breath starts the whole procedure, initiated from deep down in the diaphragm area and inhaled through the nose. You hold this deep breath up to 8 seconds. As you slowly exhale through pursed lips, formulate the pictures and affirmations: "wider-longer-warmer-heavier . . . wider-longer-warmer-heavier."

Take about 16 seconds to slowly exhale and static stretch with these pictures and affirmations. Finally, as the stretch is slowly released and the muscle is relaxed, begin another deep 8-count inhalation.

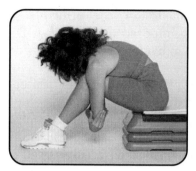

**Figure 4.26** Back Stretch. Sit on the end of the bench with your feet together on the floor. Bend over, resting your chest on thighs. Reach under legs with arms, grasp the opposite elbow, and pull both elbows together. Hold.

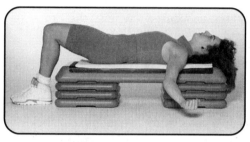

**Figure 4.27** Pectoral Stretch. Lie down on the platform with head and buttocks both comfortably on bench. Press the low back into the bench and place arms out wide to the sides, shoulder level, palms up. Relax arms as their weight falls toward the floor. Hold.

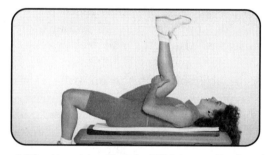

**Figure 4.28** Hamstring Stretch. Still lying on the bench, extend the left leg straight out along the platform and place foot flat on floor. Grasp behind the right thigh and gently pull the right leg toward the chest. Hold.

**Ankle Circling:** During the hamstring stretch, slowly circle the foot in all directions. Alternate with left leg and foot.

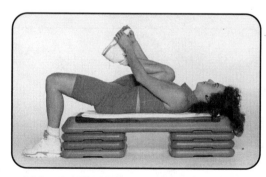

**Figure 4.29** Achilles/Calf Stretch. From the hamstring stretch, pull right knee to chest. Grasp right toes with the hands, and gently pull. Hold. Alternate with left leg and foot.

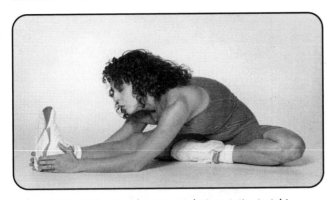

**Figure 4.30** Relaxation beginning during static stretching.

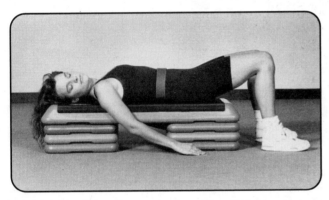

**Figure 4.31** Relaxation continuing when stretching is completed

To match pictures and affirmations with the PNF stretching, mentally take apart the muscular actions and the timeframe suggested for each portion. Do exhalation breathing during both the contract and stretch phases.

# SUMMARY

The basic principles for each segment of a step aerobics workout session are:

### WARM-UP

▌ Active, rhythmic, limbering moves
▌ Slow, standing, static stretching
▌ Proper breathing techniques throughout

### STEP AEROBICS

▌ Pre-aerobic/transitional progression from low to high
▌ Aerobic phase
▌ Post-aerobic cool-down

### STRENGTH TRAINING/MUSCLE CONDITIONING

▌ Emphasis on isolated muscle groups — chest, arms, abdominals, buttocks
▌ Weights, resistance bands and tubing, and bench exercises added

### COOL-DOWN, FLEXIBILITY, AND RELAXATION TECHNIQUES

▌ Gradual cool-down moves
▌ Flexibility training using static and PNF stretching
▌ Relaxation techniques during stretching.

Adhering to this step training workout format (for further clarity, see Table 4.1) provides you with a fun, safe, efficient, and complete session. If you prioritize this type of total physical fitness program into your schedule for a minimum of 3 days per week, you will have an excellent means of initially obtaining, and then maintaining, your fitness for a lifetime.

**TABLE 4.1  Step Training Class Overview**

| | Class Segments | | | | | | |
|---|---|---|---|---|---|---|---|
| | **Warm-up** | **Pre-Aerobic** | **Aerobic** | **Post-Aerobic** | **Strength Training** | **Stretching** | **Relaxation** |
| **Purpose of Class Segment** | Prepare muscles and joints; increase body temperature; increase blood flow; increase heart rate and lower risk of injury | Prepare cardiovascular system for the aerobic segment. Gradually raise heart rate; increase blood flow and increase oxygen to muscles | Strengthen cardiovascular system; lower body fat/body weight; decrease stress; increase energy level; improve cholesterol and blood pressure values. | Gradually lower heart rate; lower blood flow and lower blood pressure; avoid blood pooling in the legs, and dizziness | Improve muscular strength and endurance; improve muscle tone or muscle firmness | Increase flexibility; decrease muscle stiffness; relaxes the muscles | Release all muscle tension. |
| **Time/Duration** | 10–12 minutes | 4–5 minutes | 20–30 minutes | 4–5 minutes | 10–15 minutes | 5–6 minutes | 1–3 minutes |
| **Types of Moves** | Low to moderate intensity; low impact; easy to follow; static and dynamic stretches | Low increasing to moderate intensity, low impact and traveling movements | Moderate to high intensity; low and high impact; power and traveling movements | Moderate gradually decreasing to low intensity; low impact | Movements that provide resistance to the muscles using the body, bench or other equipment; slow, controlled, full range of motion movements | Static stretches; perform one stretch for each major muscle group | None. Only mental imagining (requiring no muscle movement) |
| **Tempo/speed of music (musical beats per minute, bpm)** | Tempo: 133–138 bpm | Tempo: 118–124 bpm | Tempo: 122–126 bpm | Tempo: 120–124 bpm | Tempo: 110–130 bpm; use double counts for music above 120 bpm | Tempo: less than 100 bpm | All much less than 100 bpm. Varies totally with music choice |
| **Special Instructions** | Include dynamic moves between stretches and when stretching (e.g. perform bicep curls when holding a calf stretch) to keep heart rate and body temperature high. Step classes use the step as a prop and for stretches. Do not perform basic steps above 126 bpm. Include a stretch for the upper and lower back, chest, inner thighs, hamstrings, calves and quadriceps/hip flexors. | Perform complex or advanced moves that will be used during the higher intensity step aerobic segment | Basic steps and step movements may be combined. Consider the following: •traveling movements to form patterns (A step, T step, L step, etc.) •Add-ons (moves are performed and repeated at the other side of the step). •Class formations (class is arranged in lines, circles, etc.). | Decrease use of arm movements at and above shoulder level. Can include standing muscular conditioning exercises (keep the feet moving). Can include static stretches at the very end. | Work opposing muscle groups. Use resistive equipment such as hand weights and tubing. Use the step as a prop. | Hold upper body stretches 6–15 seconds. Hold lower body stretches 10–20 seconds. Include a stretch for the neck, triceps, chest, upper and lower back, abdominals, inner thighs, quadriceps, hip flexors, and hamstrings | Sitting and/or lying on bench, or floor beside bench. |

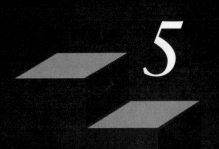

# STEP BY STEP: STEP TECHNIQUE

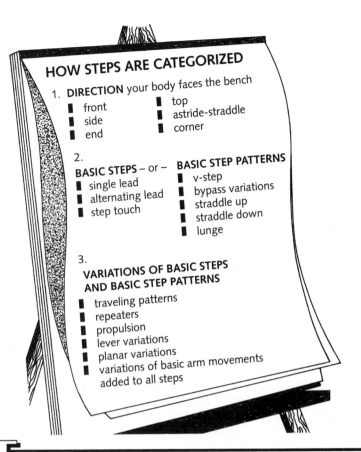

**HOW STEPS ARE CATEGORIZED**

1. **DIRECTION** your body faces the bench
   - front
   - side
   - end
   - top
   - astride-straddle
   - corner

2. **BASIC STEPS** – or – **BASIC STEP PATTERNS**
   - single lead
   - alternating lead
   - step touch
   - v-step
   - bypass variations
   - straddle up
   - straddle down
   - lunge

3. **VARIATIONS OF BASIC STEPS AND BASIC STEP PATTERNS**
   - traveling patterns
   - repeaters
   - propulsion
   - lever variations
   - planar variations
   - variations of basic arm movements added to all steps

The step aerobic techniques in this chapter represent movement depicting

- Directional approaches and orientations (your body in relation to the bench)
- Basic steps
- Basic step patterns
- Variations possible, using basic steps and basic step patterns

These step techniques are photographed and described by the mirroring technique for all *front* views shown (actual left of model is your right). Natural photography is used and described for all *side* and *rear* views. The words and the movements, therefore, are to be performed *exactly* as shown.

If you're following the movements of an instructor, position the bench for maximum visibility.

## ◼ Bench/Step Directional Approaches and Orientations[1]

Initial movement onto the bench (the direction in which your body faces the bench) can begin from the front, the end, the side, the top, astride/straddle, or corner. These are depicted in Figures 5.1 through 5.8.

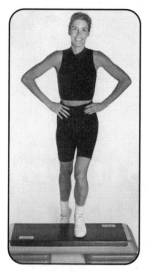

**Figure 5.1** From the **front facing the bench** squarely.

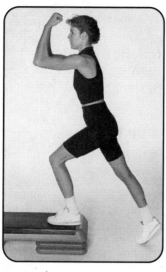

**Figure 5.2** From the **end facing the end** of the bench, step up and down.

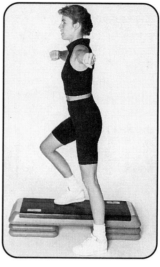

**Figure 5.3** From the **side to bench's side**.

Standing with **your side** next to the bench's **side**, step up with the foot that is closest to the side of the bench.

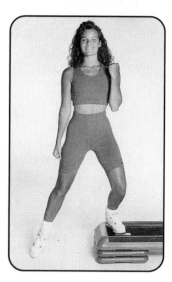

**Figure 5.4** From the **side to bench's end**.

Standing with **your side** next to the **end** of the bench, step up with the foot that is closest to the side of the bench.

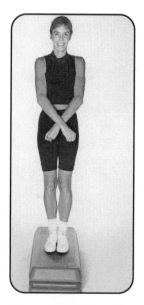

**Figure 5.5** From the **top**, in the middle of bench **facing an end**.

Standing in the middle of the bench, step off the side of the bench in a straddle position.

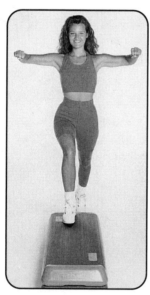

**Figure 5.6** From the **top**, at the back end of bench.

Atop, standing at the **back end of the bench**, step off the back in a forward/backward stride.

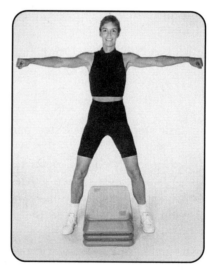

**Figure 5.7 Astride/straddle** orientation **facing bench end**.

Facing the bench's **end**, standing astride or straddle position, with bench between feet, step up onto the bench.

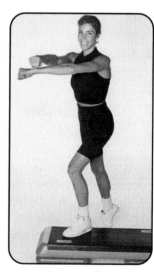

**Figure 5.8 Corner** orientation, **facing the corner**.

Facing on an **angle** toward the bench's corner; if facing at an angle to left, step up with right foot first, and if facing at an angle to right, step up with left foot first.

## ◾ Basic Steps

Three basic steps may be performed using a variety of directional approaches/orientations. They are identified as:

1. **Single lead step**
2. **Alternate lead step** — the right and left foot both serve as the lead foot *alternately initiating every 4 counts*, requiring a complete cycle for the alternating patterns to take *8 counts* (both the right foot and then left foot lead a 4-count portion of the cycle)
3. **Step touch,** performed by "touching" the *same* toe or heel on the floor or bench or by *alternating* legs. Step touch moves are often used during the warm-up segment to familiarize you with the bench, or as transition moves during the aerobic segment.

### Single Lead Step

In the single lead step, the same foot leads every 4-count cycle. For both safety and variety when using single lead step, 4-count cycle patterns, lead with the right foot for a *maximum of 1 minute,* then change to a left-foot lead. To accomplish this change in lead foot (for single cycle 4-count step patterns), perform a *non-weight-bearing, transitional, hold/touch/tap/heel* move as the last step of the cycle, initiating the change with that foot. Figures 5.9 and 5.10 depict the single lead step.

### Alternating Lead Step

You may alternate the lead leg with a bench tap up (on bench) or a floor tap down (on floor). Figures 5.11 through 5.14 show the bench approach from the front. The step also can be done from the top, end, and straddle/aside.

### Step Touch

Two basic step touches are done with the toe (Figure 5.15) and with the heel (Figure 5.16). The bench can be approached from the front (as shown in the figures), the top, the end, and straddle/astride.

## ◾ Basic Step Patterns[2]

Basic step patterns may be performed as single lead steps (4-count pattern) or alternating lead steps (8-count pattern). When performing a *single lead basic step pattern*, the *fourth count* of the cycle is weight-bearing. When executing *alternating lead steps*, there are two options:

1. When the first 3 steps are weight-bearing, the 4th is *non-weight bearing.*
2. When the first 3 steps contain a bypass move, the 4th step is *weight-bearing.*

**NOTE:** Within the descriptions in the figures in this chapter, only the moves in **BOLD** are illustrated.

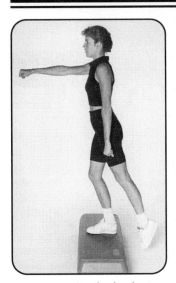

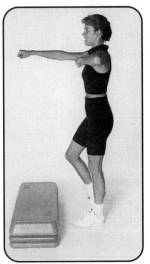

**Figure 5.9** Single lead step, up.

**Figure 5.10** Single lead step, down.

**Bench Approach:** Front (shown), top, end, and straddle/astride.

|  | R | L | R | L |  |
| --- | --- | --- | --- | --- | --- |
| Right Lead: | **Up** | up | down | **down** | 4 counts |

|  | L | R | L | R |  |
| --- | --- | --- | --- | --- | --- |
| Left Lead: | Up | up | down | down | **4 counts** |

**Arms shown:** Long-lever punching on up, up; pull, punch, on the down, down.

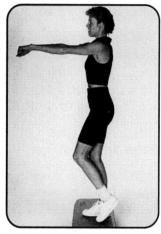

```
R      L    L      R
Up  bench tap  down  down
```

Alternate: Up (L), bench tap (R), down (R), down (L).

**8 counts**

**Arms shown:** Forward punching.

**Figure 5.11** Alternating lead step — bench tap.

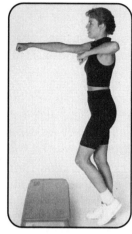

```
R      L     R       L
Up    up   down   floor tap
```

Alternate: Up (L), up (R), down (L), floor tap (R).

**8 counts**

**Arms shown:** Opposite-arm long-lever punching; same arm flexing; elbows kept shoulder high.

**Figure 5.12** Alternating step — floor tap.

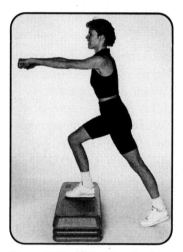

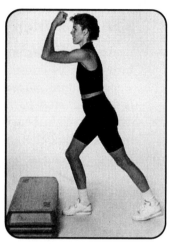

**Note:** The floor tap may also be a non-weight-bearing lunge back from the top of the step.

```
R     L      R         L
Up   up   down   down and back
```

Alternate, starting with the (L) Up.

**8 counts**.

**Arms shown:** Arms punching forward and parallel on up, up; bicep curls keeping elbows still high on the down, down.

**Figure 5.13** Alternating lead step — lunge back.

**Figure 5.14** Alternating lead step — lunge back.

```
          R          R
Bench tap  with toe   down;
repeat with left foot.
```

**4 counts**

**Arms shown:** Elbows shoulder-high, fists together on tap; fists apart on down.

**Note:** Weight-bearing leg is on the floor, not on the step.

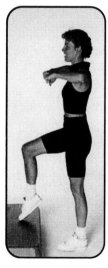

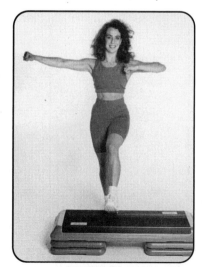

```
          R           R
Bench tap  with heel   down;
repeat with left foot.
```

**4 counts**

**Arms shown:** Arms extended to the side at shoulder level, alternating punching to the side.

**Figure 5.15** Step touch with toe.    **Figure 5.16** Step touch with heel.

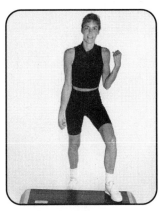

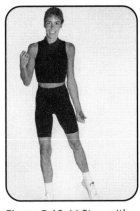

**Figure 5.17** V-Step.

**Figure 5.18** V-Step with bicep curl.

### V-Step

The bench approach is from the **front**.

| R | L | R | L |
|---|---|---|---|
| **Up-wide** | up-wide | **down-center** | down-center |

Usually cued: "out" "out" "in" "in".

**Arms shown:** Same-side single bicep curls.

## Bypass Variations

Bypass variations are shown in Figure 5.19 through 5.24. The approach can be from the **front** (shown in most of figures), side, the top, the end, astride/straddle or the corner.

### Knee-Up Bypass

| L | R |
|---|---|
| Up, | **knee lift** |

(bypasses the bench and lifts)

R
down (to floor)

L
down (to floor)

**Arms shown:** Initiate from arms fully extended to the sides, shoulder high with palms up: single short-lever curls on the up and knee lift; return one at a time to the long-lever, shoulder-high initial position on the down, down.

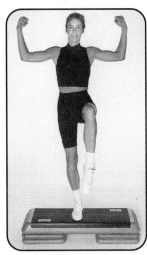

**Figure 5.19** Knee-up bypass.

### Kick-Forward Bypass

| L | R | R | L |
|---|---|---|---|
| Up | **kick forward** | down (to floor) | down (to floor) |

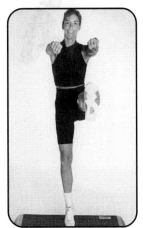

**Arms shown:** Arms sweep up from sides, together and parallel on up, kick; sweep together and parallel back down to sides on the down, down.

**Figure 5.20** Kick-forward bypass.

### Kick-Back Bypass

| L | R | |
|---|---|---|
| Up | **kick back** | (a "**long lever** raising" motion) |

R
down (to floor)

L
down (to floor)

**Arms shown:** Initiate from arms fully extended down at sides: Raise same (one) elbow out wide to shoulder high with fist ending at waist for the up and kick back; lower to initial position at side with each down, down.

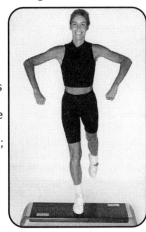

**Figure 5.21** Kick-back bypass.

## Side Leg Lift Bypass

L    R
Up  **side leg lift**  (a knee pointing forward position),

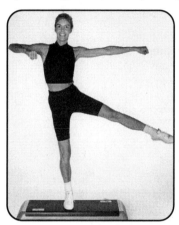

        R
     down (to floor)
        L
     down (to floor)

**Arms shown:** Both arms raised simultaneously to bent-arm lateral raise position for up; same arm (one) extends out to side shoulder high for the side leg lift; extended arm returns to bent-arm lateral raise on the down; both arms lowered simultaneously on the last down.

**Figure 5.22** Side leg lift bypass.

## Adductor Bypass

R      L
Up  **lift heel to front**
(a **short-lever** raising motion)

     L
  down (to floor)

     R
  down (to floor)

**Arms shown:** Both arms extend to side at shoulder level when you step up. As the heel lifts to the front, the opposite hand touches the instep; when you step down, the arms lower to the side.

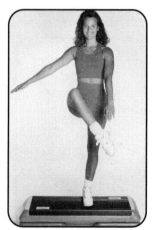

**Figure 5.23** Adductor bypass.

## Hamstring Curl Bypass

R      L
Up  **lift heel to back**
**short-lever** raising motion)

     L
   down (to floor)

     R
   down (to floor)

**Arms shown:** Both arms extend to side at shoulder level when you step up. As the heel lifts to the back, the opposite hand reaches back and touches the heel; when you step down, the arms lower to the side.

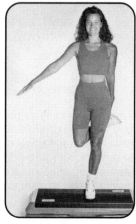

**Figure 5.24** Hamstring curl bypass.

## Straddle Up

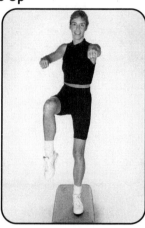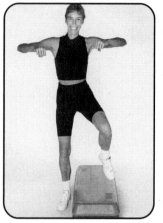

**Figure 5.25–5.26** Straddle up; with arms punching forward.

R              L
Up    knee lift (bypasses bench and lifts waist-high),

      L              R
  straddle down (to floor)    straddle down (to floor)

Alternate pattern, stepping now up (L) and knee lifting (R), followed by the straddle down, down.

**Arms shown:** Shoulder high, short-levers, and fists together at center. Opposite arm punches forward on lift.

**Note:** For variety, try the other bypass moves shown earlier — kick forward, kickback, or side leg lift. Straddle Up can also be a non-bypass basic step pattern.

## Straddle Down

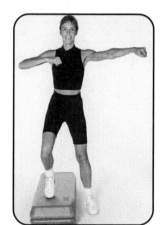

       R
   **Straddle Down**
  (on R side of bench)

       L
   **Straddle down**
  (on L side of bench)

  R        L
  up       up

**Arms shown:** Shoulder high, short-levers, and fists together at center. Same long-lever arm extends out to side as same leg steps out. One arm at a time returns back in to center on each up, up step.

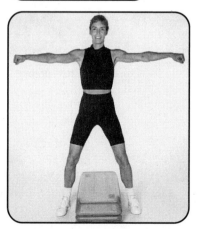

**Figure 5.27–5.28** Straddle down; with arms extended.

**Lunge (from top)**

| | L | L |
|---|---|---|
| | **Touch down side** | **up** |
| | R | R |
| | **touch down side** | **up** |

**Arms shown:** When left leg steps to the side, punch the left arm in front at an angle; when right leg steps to the side, punch the right arm in front at an angle.

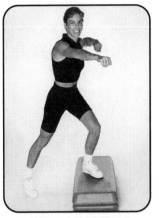 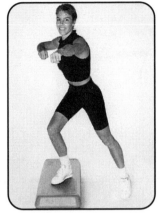

**Figure 5.29** Lunge left from **top** of bench.       **Figure 5.30** Lunge right.

**Lunge (from end)**

| | L | L |
|---|---|---|
| | Touch down back | up |
| | R | R |
| | **touch down back** | up |

**Arms shown:** Arms parallel at shoulder level; bicep-curl touch down back; and punch forward on the touch up on bench.

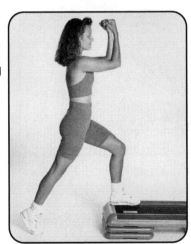

**Figure 5.31** Lunge back from **end** of bench.

## ▪▪▪ Variations of Basic Steps and Basic Step Patterns

To add interest and variety to basic steps and basic step patterns, you can implement a number of variations.[3] The following step variations can be categorized as traveling, repeaters, propulsion, lever, and planar. Creative arm movements also play a significant role in adding variety and interest to the step training workout.

## Traveling Patterns

### TURN STEP — LENGTH OF THE BENCH (Figures 5.32–5.35)

The turn step, pictured in Figures 5.32–5.35, is shown using natural photography and descriptive words, as it could not be photographed, and therefore described, from a "mirrored" perspective. Remember to keep your eyes on the platform.

**Bench Approach:** Side (shown).

Single lead – **4 counts**; Alternating lead – **8 counts**

| L | R | L | R |
|---|---|---|---|
| Up | **body 1/2 turns left and up** | down | tap down |

**Arms shown:** Shoulder-high alternating punch and pull back.

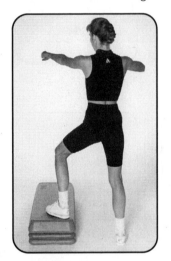 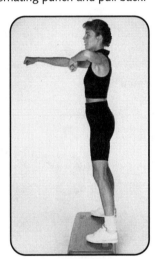

**Figure 5.32**                    **Figure 5.33**

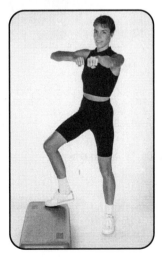 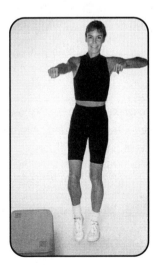

**Figure 5.34**                    **Figure 5.35**

## OVER THE TOP – WIDTH OF THE BENCH
## (Figures 5.36–5.39)

For variety on the *fourth* step, instead of tapping the floor: touch heel on the bench; knee up; or kick front.

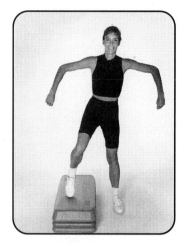

**Figure 5.36.**

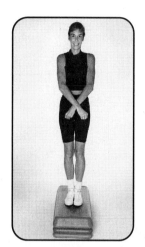

**Figure 5.37.**

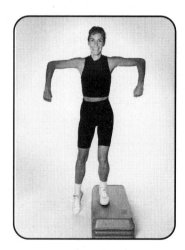

**Figure 5.38.**

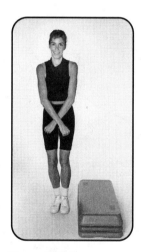

**Figure 5.39.**

**Bench Approach:** Side (shown).

Single lead – **4 counts**; Alternating lead – **8 counts**

| L | R | L | R |
|---|---|---|---|
| Up | up | down on the left side of bench/platform | touch down |

Cued: "up", "over", "down", "tap".

**Arms shown:** Elbows pointing skyward and shoulder high, with arms wide open on the first, third, fifth, and seventh steps; arms low and crossed in front on even-numbered steps.

## ACROSS THE TOP – LENGTH OF THE BENCH
## (Figures 5.40–5.43)

Arms are at shoulder level; when legs are apart, arms are straight out to the side; bend arms into the chest when feet are together.

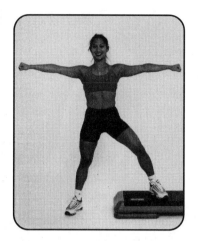

**Figure 5.40.**

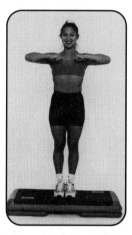

**Figure 5.41.**

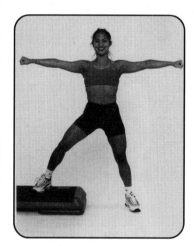

**Figure 5.42.**

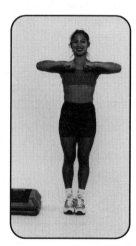

**Figure 5.43.**

**Bench Approach:** End (shown)

Single lead – **4 counts**; Alternating lead – **8 counts**

| R | L | R | L |
|---|---|---|---|
| Up | up | down on the right side of bench | touch down |

Cued: "up", "across", "down", "tap".

## CORNER TO CORNER (Figures 5.44–5.47)

For variety on the *second* and *sixth* steps, use any bypass move (knee, kick front/back, side leg lift, hamstring curl, adductor).

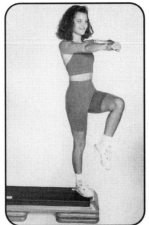

Figure 5.44.

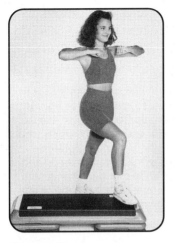

Figure 5.45.

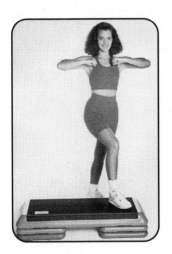

Figure 5.46.

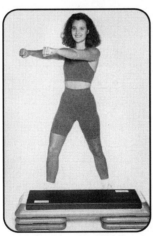

Figure 5.47.

**Bench Approach:** Corner (shown).

Alternating lead step – **8 counts**

| L | R | R | L |
|---|---|---|---|
| **Up** | **knee lift** | **down** | **down turning body on diagonal facing left corner** |

**Arms shown:** Arms at shoulder level, row position, punch the opposite arm forward as the knee comes up, pull-punch in on down, and both arms punch forward when the body turns to the diagonal.

## DIAGONAL OVER (Figures 5.48–5.51)

Because you never approach the bench with your back to it, the next steps must use either the close end of the bench, or all floor patterns, to realign your body so your front or your side faces the bench.

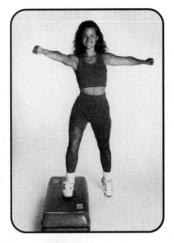

Figure 5.48.

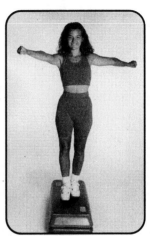

Figure 5.49.

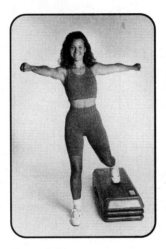

Figure 5.50.

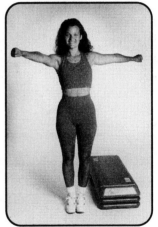

Figure 5.51.

**Bench Approach:** Side (shown).

Single lead step – **4 counts.**

| L | R | L | R |
|---|---|---|---|
| **Up-forward** | **up** | **down-forward** | **down** |

Cued: "up", "to the middle", "down", "tap".

**Arms shown:**
Arms to the side at shoulder level, and angled in the direction the body is traveling.

## AROUND THE CORNER (Figures 5.52–5.54)

This variation uses natural photography, as it is a traveling sequence that can't be mirrored.

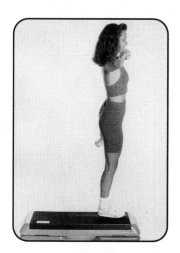

Figure 5.52.

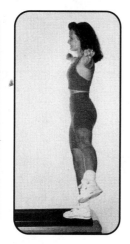

Figure 5.53.

Figure 5.54.

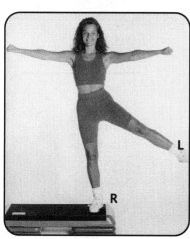

**Bench Approach:** Side (shown).

Single lead step, 3 cycles each – **4 counts.**

| R | L | L | R |
|---|---|---|---|
| Up | side leg lift | down (to floor) | tap (on floor) |

Repeat from the **end** (Figure 5.53) and on the **other side** (Figure 5.54) of the bench.

**Arms shown:** Both arms raised to the side when the leg lifts to the side, and lowered when stepping down to the floor.

## Repeaters

Repeaters are illustrated in Figures 5.55–5.57. For variety, instead of taps use knee lifts, forward kicks, kick backs, side leg lifts and so on.

This step may be a single or an alternating lead step; however, keep the number of repeaters limited to maximum of 4. A repeater is when any *non-weight-bearing phase of a move is repeated.*

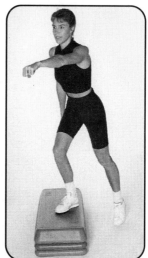

For example: Using a diagonal front approach, **step up (L), tap up (R), tap down and back (R)**, tap up (R), tap down and back (R), tap up (R), step down (R), step down (L) and turn to face the other corner. Alternate stepping up (R) and tapping (L).

Figure 5.55.

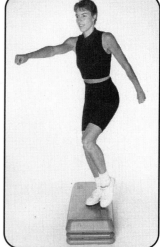

Figure 5.56.

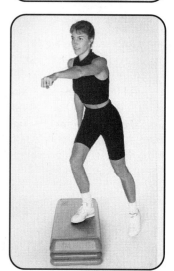

Figure 5.57.

## Propulsion Steps

Both feet push off the ground or bench, exchanging positions during the airborne phase of the pattern. Propulsion steps are commonly used with lunge steps. A sample propulsion step pattern is shown in Figures 5.58 and 5.59. Propulsion moves also may be used when performing bypass or traveling moves by adding a hop or pushing off the foot on the bench (Figures 5.60 and 5.61).

## Lever Variations

Lever refers to the joint that initiates the movement. Thus, arm or leg movements may be classified as long- or short-lever movements and can be varied as such. Short-lever moves include knee lifts and bicep curls (Figure 5.62), and long-lever moves include kicks and deltoid raises (Figure 5.63).

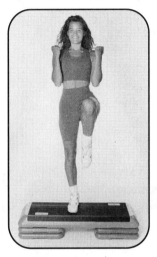

**Figure 5.62** Short-levers.

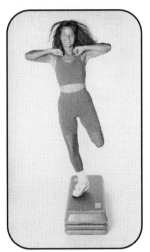 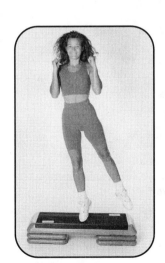

**Figure 5.58.**      **Figure 5.59.**
Propulsion lunges.

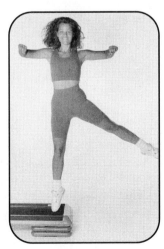 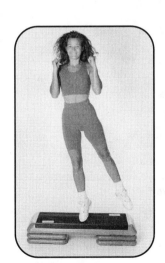

**Figure 5.60** Bypass.      **Figure 5.61** Across the top.

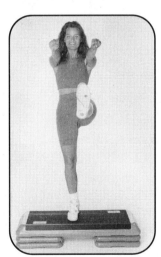

**Figure 5.63** Long-levers.

## Planar Variations

The body can be divided into three different planes: frontal, transverse, and sagittal (Figure 5.64). As an element of variation, planar changes refer to the space in which the arms or legs, or both, are moving around the body.[4]

One way to modify a bypass move, such as a kick front or knee lift in the *frontal plane* (Figures 5.65 and 5.66), would be with a bypass side leg lift or a propulsion lunge in the *sagittal plane* (Figures 5.67 and 5.68).

To vary a move in the *transverse plane*, simply keep the same leg movement and vary the arms, or keep the same arm movement and vary the legs.

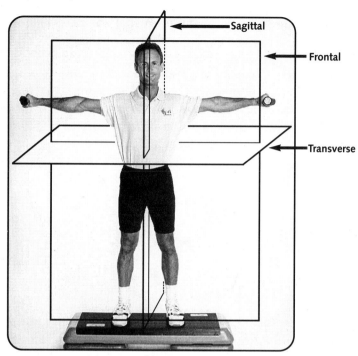

**Figure 5.64**  Three planes of body.

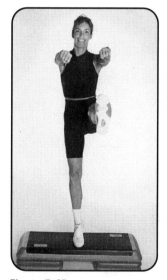
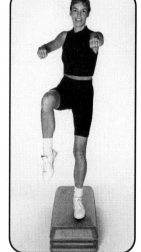
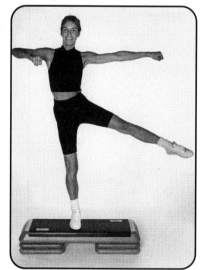
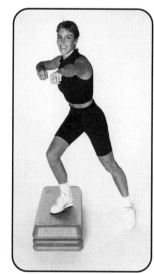

**Figure 5.65**  **Figure 5.66**
**Frontal Plane**

**Figure 5.67**  **Figure 5.68**
**Sagittal Plane**

## ■ Variations of Basic Arm Movements

Variations of basic steps and basic step patterns include variations in arm movements. Varying the arm movements adds *significantly* to the variety of your work-out. Before adding any arm movements, however, be sure you are comfortable with the basic steps and basic step patterns. Then progress gradually with the easier and less intense versions of the following variations. When the steps are safely mastered, add the more difficult and intense arm movements.

## Bilateral/Unilateral Arm Movements

Bilateral moves refer to movements that are performed in unison or both arms doing the same action (Figure 5.69). These are easier than unilateral movements. Unilateral refers to performing moves in which each arm or leg is doing something different (Figure 5.70). This is more difficult.

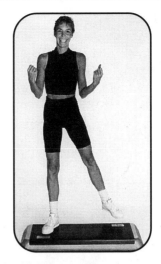 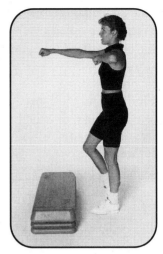

**Figure 5.69.** Bilateral movement.

**Figure 5.70.** Unilateral movement.

## Complementary/ Opposition Movements

Complementary moves refer to coordinating arm and leg movements. For example, when the left leg moves, the left arm moves, and when the right leg moves the right arm moves (Figure 5.71). This is relatively easy.

Opposition moves are naturally flowing and help you maintain balance but psychologically are usually more challenging when step training. An opposition move is one in which the left arm moves with the right leg and the right arm moves with the left leg (Figure 5.72).

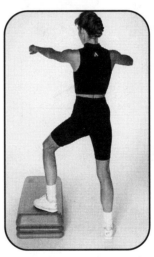 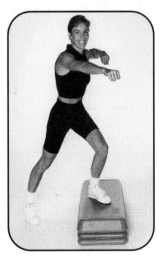

**Figure 5.71.** Complementary movement.

**Figure 5.72.** Opposition movement.

## Low-/Middle-/Upper-Range Arm Movements

Start with the less intense, low-range motions (elbows kept low, near your waist). Gradually incorporate more intense, middle-range motions (elbows are chest-to-shoulder high). Finally, you can progress to the highly intense upper-range arm movements (elbows are at and above shoulder level).

## LOW-RANGE (ELBOW) ARM MOVEMENTS

Figures 5.73–5.80 illustrate low-range (elbow) movements. These include Bicep Curls, Hammer Curls, Low Wide 'n Cross, Row Low, and Triceps Kick-Backs.

### Bicep Curls

With elbows **fixed** at the sides, **palms up** (Figure 5.73), flex both elbows, forearms moving toward shoulders (Figure 5.74). For **Alternating Bicep Curls**, alternate the right and left forearms (Figure 5.75).

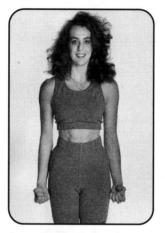

**Figure 5.73**   Bicep Curl.

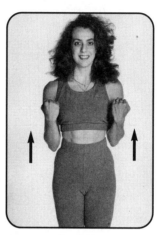

**Figure 5.74**   Bicep Curls, arms moving up.

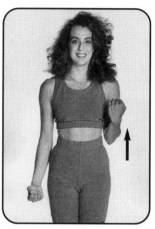

**Figure 5.75**   Bicep Curls, alternating forearms.

### Hammer Curls

With elbows **fixed** at the sides and **palms facing** each other, flex both elbows, forearms toward the shoulders (Figure 5.76).

### Alternating Hammer Curls:

Alternate the right and left forearms (Figure 5.77).

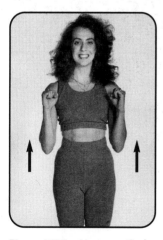
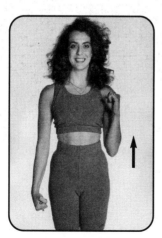

**Figure 5.76**   Hammer Curl.     **Figure 5.77**   Alternating Hammer Curl.

### Low Wide 'n Cross

With the elbows at the sides and forearms wide (Figure 5.78), criss-cross the arms at waist level in front of the body, keeping palms up.

By rotating both elbows forward, **Low Punches** can be performed by extending both elbows forward, away from the body (palms still up), or **Alternating Low Punches**, by extending one forearm at a time.

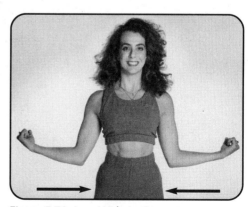

**Figure 5.78** Low Wide 'n Cross.

## Row Low

Begin with forearms (only) extended in front of body, waist-level. Pull the elbows backward (Figure 5.79) until the fists are next to the waist. Return to starting position.

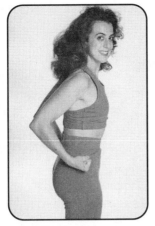

**Figure 5.79** Row Low.

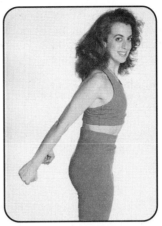

**Figure 5.80** Tricep Kick Back.

## Tricep Kick Backs

With the elbows **fixed** behind the shoulders and fists next to sides (Figure 5.79), extend both elbows, forearms moving backward (Figure 5.80).

For **Alternating Tricep Kick Backs**, alternate right and left arms. Palms can face up/in/down.

## MID-RANGE ARM MOVEMENTS

Mid-range arm movements shown here are the Criss-Crossover, Double and Single Side-Outs, Front Shoulder Raises, Shoulder Punch, Side Lateral Raise, Upright Row, and Cross and Lateral Raise.

## Double Side-Out

Begin with fists under chin at shoulder level, palms down, elbows directly out (Figure 5.83). Extend both arms wide out to the sides, keeping elbows at shoulder height. Pull the fists back into the chin.

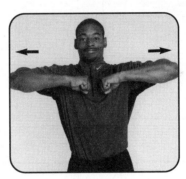

**Figure 5.83** Double side-out.

## Criss-Crossovers

Keeping elbows at chest height, criss-cross the arms over each other, palms facing down (Figure 5.81).

Alternate the arm that crosses over the top, for each repetition (Figure 5.82).

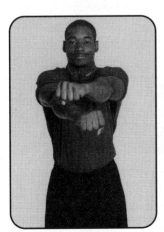

**Figure 5.81** Criss-Crossover.

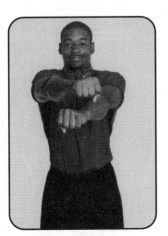

**Figure 5.82** Criss-Crossover alternating arms.

## Single Side-Outs

Alternate the right and left arms (Figure 5.84).

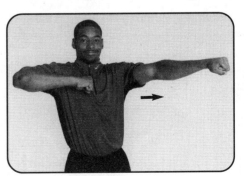

**Figure 5.84** Single side-out.

## Front Shoulder Raise

Begin with the palms together in front of the thighs. Keeping elbows soft, raise both arms straight up to the front to shoulder level, palms down (Figure 5.85).

Alternate right and left arms, for **Alternating Front Shoulder Raise** (Figure 5.86).

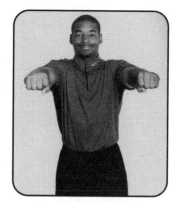

**Figure 5.85** Front shoulder raise.

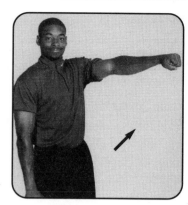

**Figure 5.86** Alternating front shoulder raise.

## Shoulder Punch

Start with the hands lightly resting on the shoulders. Extend one arm forward (Figure 5.87), or diagonally across the body, at shoulder height. Pull back and return to shoulder.

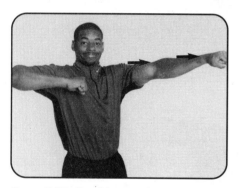

**Figure 5.87** Shoulder punch.

## Side Lateral Raise

Start with the fists together in front of the thighs. Lift arms up and out wide, palms facing down, always leading with the elbows, keeping them slightly bent (Figure 5.88).

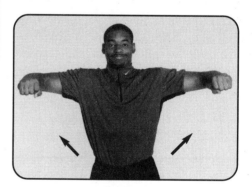

**Figure 5.88** Side lateral raise.

## Upright Row

Begin with the palms in front of the thighs (Figure 5.89). Keeping the fists close to the body and elbows wide, raise the hands up to chin (Figure 5.90).

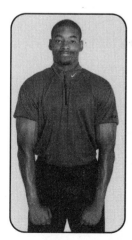
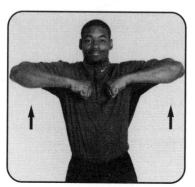

**Figure 5.89–5.90** Upright row; raising hands.

## Cross and Lateral Raise

Begin with arms crossed low in front of abdomen, palms facing body (Figures 5.91). Uncross palms and laterally raise elbows up pointing skyward to shoulder height, keeping arms wide open (Figure 5.92).

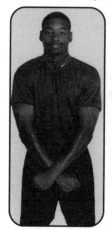
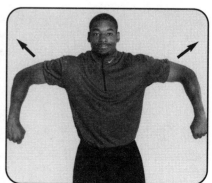

**Figure 5-91–5.92** Cross and lateral raise.

## UPPER-RANGE ARM MOVEMENTS

Upper-range arm movements include the Side-L, Front-L, Overhead Press, Triceps Extension, Slice, and Butterflies.

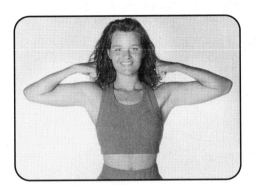

**Figure 5.93** Side-L.

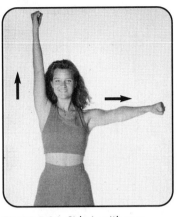

**Figure 5.94** Side L with arm movements.

### Side-L

Begin with fists resting on shoulders (Figures 5.93). Simultaneously extend one arm straight out to side at shoulder height while extending the other arm upward above the head (Figure 5.94). Pull both fists back to shoulders and repeat, other direction.

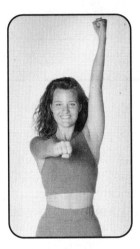

**Figure 5.95** Front-L.

### Front-L

Start with fists resting on shoulders (see Figure 5.93). Simultaneously extend one arm straight out in front of you, shoulder height, while extending other arm upward above the head (Figure 5.95). Pull both fists back to shoulders and repeat, other direction.

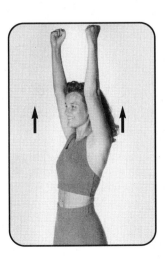

**Figure 5.96** Overhead press.

### Overhead Press

Start with fists resting on shoulders (see Figure 5.93). With palms facing, extend arms upward over head, keeping elbows close to ears (Figure 5.96).

For **Alternating Overhead Press**, alternate the right and left arms.

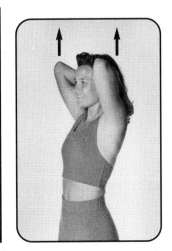

**Figure 5.97** Triceps extension.

### Triceps Extension

Begin with elbows fixed high, near ears, and fists on shoulders (Figure 5.97). With palms facing, extend arms high and parallel overhead (see Figure 5.96).

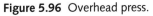

## Slice

Begin with fists facing and resting on shoulders, elbows low at sides (Figure 5.98). Simultaneously extend one arm upward straight above head while extending the other arm downward, along side of the leg (Figure 5.99). Pull both fists back to shoulders, and repeat with other side high/low.

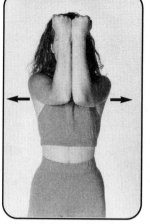

**Figure 5.100**  Butterflies.

## Butterflies

Begin with fists and forearms together and parallel in front of face, elbows pointing down (Figure 5.100). Keeping elbows shoulder-high, open them wide and out to the sides (Figure 5.101.

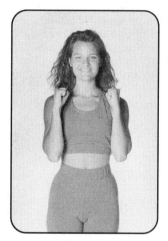

**Figure 5.98**  Slice.

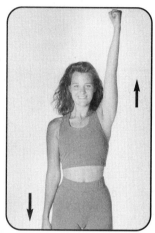

**Figure 5.99**  Slice showing upward arm movement.

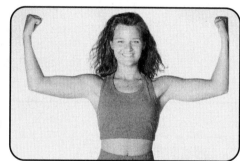

**Figure 5.101** Butterflies showing arm movement.

## SUMMARY

Techniques illustrating the fundamentals of step training presented in this chapter include:

▌ Ways to approach the bench

▌ The basic steps and basic step patterns

▌ Techniques for adding variety to the basic step movements.

As you advance in your fitness and stepping skills, adding *variety* will become your next challenge, by developing more intricate foot patterns and by adding many powerful arm movements, taken primarily from strength training principles. Chapter 6, details the principles of creatively putting moves together to a beat.

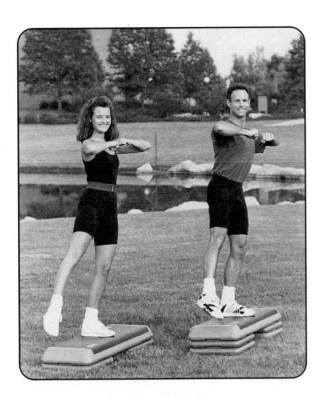

Step training involves stepping on, off, over, and around the bench while doing a series of movements to music. Outside, inside, in a class setting with a group, on a trip, alone at home — the location is your choice. The moves range from simple basic steps to more complex basic step patterns. Once the basic steps and basic step patterns are mastered, they may be put together to create a variety of challenging patterns and combinations.

Whether you are a beginner or an advanced stepper, once you have mastered the basic steps and step patterns, you will be able to put them together to develop a challenging and safe personalized fitness program to help you reach your goals. If you are beginning, you may find it a challenge determining how much or what exercises to do. Start slowly and progress at your own pace. Your personal step training program will be determined by your fitness level and what you want to accomplish. Now you are ready to put step moves together to achieve your goals!

## ■■■ Recipe for Success

Putting step aerobic movements together can be compared metaphorically to making a classic, time-honored recipe. A recipe requires three things to achieve the same excellent results that can be duplicated again and again by anyone:

1. The *ingredients* (key components)
2. The *amounts* of each ingredient
3. The *order* in which they are best used.

Combining movement, too, requires key ingredients or basic components for a balanced program, the amounts or numbers of movement possibilities and repetitions of those moves, and the order of their importance (methodology). This constitutes the recipe or blueprint for consistent success. With an understanding of these three factors, you can become the creative source of your own personal program, or for use when you are placed in the leadership role of directing others.

In step training, exercise movements are planned around the following three key ingredients:[1]

- *Biomechanical safety,* to avoid injuries
- *Physiological considerations,* to consistently achieve the overall training effect and other individual fitness goals
- *Psychological considerations,* to achieve short-term, present-moment enjoyment and long-term enjoyment for adherence to the program.

These ingredients must be factored into your planning and then expressed, moment-by-moment, as directed creative movement.

*Transition* means the flow from one movement to the next. When designing combinations and patterns, transitions are necessary to develop balanced combinations. In step training, as in aerobics, some moves easily follow one another. Table 6.1 lists basic moves and basic step patterns that "go together."[2]

## ■ Combining Movements

The two basic ways to put individual step training moves together are linear progressions and repeating progressions. Each can meet the challenge of keeping fun in your fitness pursuits.

## Linear Progressions

Linear movements consist of consecutive repetitions — one following another, then another, and so on. Linear progressions are used to introduce new moves, add variations, gradually increase intensity, and "build" sequences.[3]

Start with one basic move or basic step pattern, and change one element at a time. For example, using an alternating lead turn-step (length of the bench) (Figures 5.32–5.35), change one element (arms, legs, intensity) at a time. As possibilities for change, instead of a **tap down** (Figure 6.1), perform a **lunge back** (Figure 6.2), a **knee up** (Figure 6.3), or a **chest press** (Figure 6.4).

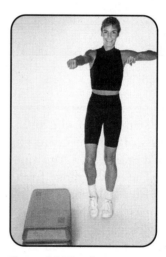
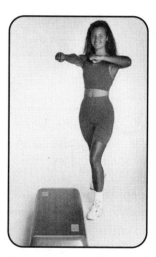

**Figure 6.1** Tap down.          **Figure 6.2** Lunge back (vary legs).

## TABLE 6.1   Ways to Combine Step Movements

| Basic Step to: | Knee Up to: | Tap Step to: | Turn Step to: | Over the Top to: | Straddle Down to: | Straddle Up to: |
|---|---|---|---|---|---|---|
| Knee up | Traveling knee up | Knee up | Tap down | Tap down | Over the top | Repeaters |
| Tap up | Basic step | Traveling knee up | Over the top | Turn step | Lunge | Tap down |
| V-step | Repeaters | Turn step | Straddle down | | Tap ups | Over the top |
| Repeaters | | Repeaters | | | Astride | |

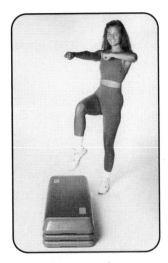

**Figure 6.3** Knee up (vary legs).

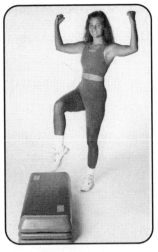

**Figure 6.4** Chest press (vary arms).

## Repeating Progressions

The second way of putting moves together is a building-block method called repeating progressions. These are a series of movements combined to form a specific combination. By beginning with a basic step move or basic step pattern, then adding another and putting them together, you create a combination.

You should start simply; gradually develop 4- and 8-count patterns, and piece them together. One advantage to this method is that is allows you to relax and anticipate what will happen next.

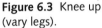 **Step Training Variations**

The underlying structure of an effective step training program has been established. It can be exciting now to build upon that basic success strategy by adding appropriate change or variation to your program. The following list identifies some of the reasons you'll want to include variety:

- progression from the status of beginner to intermediate, or intermediate to advanced, in both aerobic capacity and motor skill level;
- biomechanical needs (such as rehabilitation from injury)
- physiological needs (such as varying the intensity or resuming after an illness)
- psychological needs (such as increasing the difficulty of a workout to keep you continually mentally and physically challenged by using advanced movements or increasing step height, or both.

## Advanced Step Movements

Advanced step patterns[3,4,5] utilize various bench orientation/approaches and can be challenging because of the changes in the lead leg and weight-bearing leg.

### L-STEP (Figures 6.5–6.8)

Directional approach: from the front.

| L | R | R | L |
|---|---|---|---|
| Up | tap up | down side | down tap |
| L | R | R | L |
| Up | tap up | down back | down |
| | | | (step out wide to other side) |

Repeat on other side.

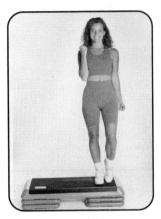

**Figure 6.5** L-Step: R tap up.

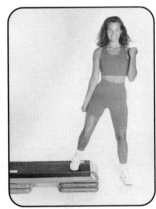

**Figure 6.6** L-Step: R down side.

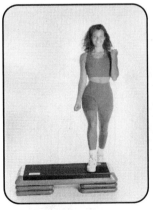

**Figure 6.7** L-Step: R down back.

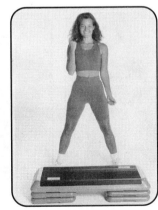

**Figure 6.8** L-Step: L down.

## BOX STEP (Figure 6.9)

Directional approach: from the side

| R | L | R | L |
|---|---|---|---|
| Outside leg up | up | down | down |

> *May progress to a single or alternating lead basic step to the front by performing a ¼ turn when the outside leg steps up.*

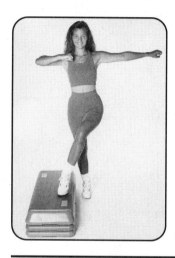

**Figure 6.9.** Outside leg up (step 1) of Box Step.

## PIVOT OVER (Figures 6.10–6.12)

Directional approach: from the side

| L | L | R | L |
|---|---|---|---|
| Up | hop ½ turn | down side | down (tap) |

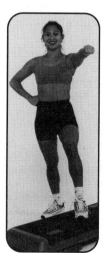 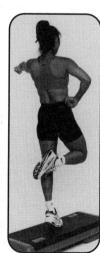 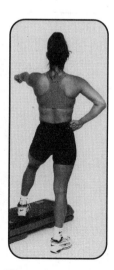

**Figure 6.10** Pivot Over (not shown as mirror image): L up.

**Figure 6.11** Pivot Over: L hop 1/2 turn.

**Figure 6.12** Pivot Over: R down side.

## SCISSOR OVER (Figures 6.13–6.15)

Directional approach: from the side

| R | L | L | R |
|---|---|---|---|
| Up | cross behind | **down** | **down** |

Repeat from the other side, stepping up with the left.

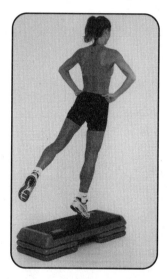

**Figure 6.13**
Scissor Over: Up R.

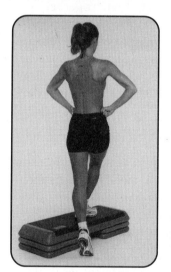 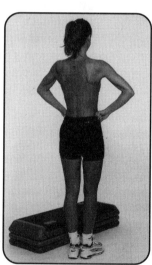

**Figure 6.14** Scissor Over: L cross behind and down R side.

**Figure 6.15** Scissor Over: Down R.

## STEP, TOUCH, STRADDLE TO OTHER SIDE (Figure 6.16)

Directional approach: from the side.

Figure 6.16 illustrates an empty bench with sequential placement location of each foot.

| R | L | L | R |
|---|---|---|---|
| Up | tap up | step down | step down |
| (1) | (2) | (3) | other side (4) |
| L | R | R | L |
| step up | tap up | step down | tap down |
| (5) | (6) | (7) | (8) |

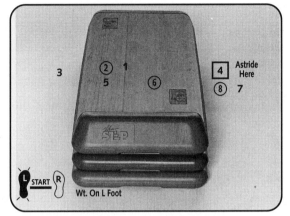

**Figure 6.16.** Bench depicting Step, Touch, Straddle to Other Side step.

## DOUBLE "T" STEP (Figure 6.17)

Directional approach: from the end.

All basic steps and basic step patterns can be used to create an 8- or a 16-count step pattern that incorporates *all three sides* of the bench, beginning from the end of the bench. When you get creative, your back should never face the bench while you are stepping up. Only three sides of the bench are available to you for any one pattern.

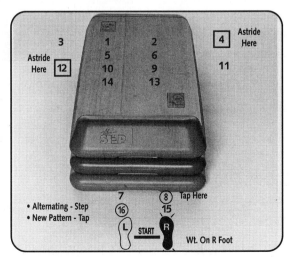

**Figure 6.17.** Bench depicting Double "T" step.

Figure 6.17 illustrates an empty bench with sequential placement location of each foot. Beginning from the bench's end and with your weight on your *right foot* on the floor, step up on bench to the #1 location with your *left foot*. Continue with the pattern, placing your next foot on top of the bench, or on the side or at the end on the floor, wherever the sequential number indicates foot placement.

> When repeating the pattern, final step #16 takes weight onto L foot. The next move is up (R).
> *When changing to create a totally new pattern, final step #16 is a non-weight-bearing move (like a tap), with the next weight-bearing step on that same (tap) foot, either in place on the floor, or up, on the bench.*

## TURN, STRADDLE, TURN (Figure 6.18)

Directional approach: from the side

Figure 6.18 illustrates an empty bench with sequential placement location of each foot. Beginning on the bench's right side, with your weight on your right foot on the floor, step up on the bench to the #1 location with your left foot (see Figures 5.32–5.34). On the fourth step, the right foot straddles the bench, facing the opposite direction. Then the left foot steps up to begin a turn step on the left side.

| L | R | L | R |
|---|---|---|---|
| Up | up | down | down straddle |
| (1) | (2) | (3) | (4) |
| L | R | L | R |
| Up | up | down | down tap |
| (5) | (6) | (7) | (8) |

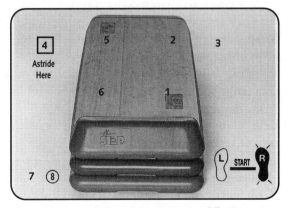

**Figure 6.18** Bench depicting a Turn, Straddle, Turn step.

## ■■■ Varying the Intensity

Step training enables you to design a program that will continually improve your overall fitness, whether you are a beginning, an intermediate, or an advanced stepper — and all within the same setting. It is simply a matter of knowing *how to adjust the intensity* of what you are doing. (Intensity, again, is directly reflected by heartbeats per minute, or rate of perceived exertion.)

As you continue to do the simple basic steps, basic step patterns, and most of the step pattern variations, you can increase or decrease the intensity to accommodate your individual needs (regarding fitness, skill, health status, or goals), by changing any of the following variables:

- Raising or lowering the bench height
- Using long- or short-levers
- Using high- or low-impact steps
- Using difficult or easy arm movement range-of-motion levels
- Increasing or decreasing the music tempo or beats per minute (not a variable the *individual* has control over in a group setting).

In the following discussion, beginners are regular exercisers who have never done step training, intermediates are regular step trainers, and advanced refers to skilled, regular step training participants.[6]

### Beginning Step Trainers

Before beginning a step training program, your fitness level must be determined as detailed in Chapter 2. Based on the results of the fitness assessment, you will have a better idea how quickly you can expect to progress by varying the intensity in your step training program.

When participating in step training for the first time, to ensure safety, select a 4" or 6" bench and concentrate on performing just the foot movements. Omit the arm patterns altogether by keeping your hands on your hips.[7]

Next glance down and watch the bench and your feet, as to where they are to move *next*. When you are comfortable with the step height and the step moves, you will be able to step safely and efficiently in the right location without constantly looking down at the bench.

If you become temporarily fatigued or cannot follow the step patterns, lower the platform or perform the moves just on the floor, until you recover your breath or timing and coordination.

### Intermediate Step Trainers

If you have regularly engaged in beginning step training and can now safely and efficiently use good form to complete a step session, consider any of the following to increase your intensity, or workload, to sustain the training zone heart rate:

- Increase step height in 2" increments (see Chapter 3);
- Increase music tempo gradually from 118 bpm to 125 bpm (see Chapter 3);
- Intensify arm movements by using a larger range-of-motion (see next section);
- Vary footwork (presented later in chapter).

Each of these variables should be added only one at a time.

### Advanced Step Trainers

From research findings conducted by fitness professionals, product literature promoting correct use of the equipment involved, and the professional experiences of both authors, the following are the *maximum safe limits* when step training:

- Bench height: 12"
- Music tempo: 128 bpm
- Step pattern variations that include high-impact (propulsion) moves: 8–16 counts of continuous repetitions, followed by low-impact steps for at least 4–8 counts, before resuming high-impact moves.
- High-range arm movements: 8 counts of continuous repetition, followed by at least 16 counts of middle- or low-range moves, before resuming high-range moves.

These maximum limits for the advanced step trainer are achieved steadily, over time, and are progressively changed or added, one at a time.

### Increasing Arm Movement Intensity

All step training arm movements are similar to those used during strength training and always must be performed in a controlled manner. Intensity can be increased *significantly* by the type of arm movements.

The joint from which the arm movement originates determines the intensity. *Long-lever* arm movements, originating from the shoulder, provide more intensity than *short-lever* moves, which originate from the elbow.

The *range-of-motion* of the arm movements directly reflects the more and less intense moves. *Low-range* moves (Figures 5.73–5.80), in which the elbows remain near the waist and sides, are the least intense. *Middle-range* moves (Figures 5.81–5.92), in which the elbows are kept at chest level, provide more intensity. *Upper-range* arm movements (Figures 5.93–5.101), in which the elbows are shoulder high and above the head, provide the most intensity and increase in workload.

Because arm movements classified as upper-range tend to escalate the heart rate higher than the accompanying work reflects, the number of upper-range movements should be limited. Enough methods to escalate intensity to challenge your workload are available without continually doing upper-range arm movements.

## Varying Footwork

Another way to modify exercise intensity is to vary specific footwork and impact. Lunge-steps, traveling movements, and repeaters create a higher intensity than other step patterns tested.[8, 9] All high-impact moves (when you are momentarily airborne and landing on one or two feet, such as propulsions) create a higher intensity compared to low-impact footwork, when at least one foot is always on the ground or bench.

## Applying Intensity Principles

The following figures illustrate how to vary (increase or decrease) the intensity of basic moves and basic step patterns[10] by varying the arm and leg levers and range-of-motion used.

## STEP TOUCH BYPASS: LOW INTENSITY (Figure 6.19)

Directional approach: corner

| L | R | R | L |
|---|---|---|---|
| Up | **tap up** | down | tap down |

(Hip joint used in low range-of-motion).
Arms: Bicep curl (low-range, short-lever)

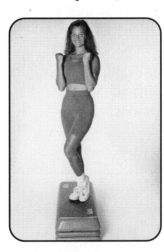

**Figure 6.19.** Step Touch Bypass: Low intensity.

## STEP TOUCH BYPASS: MODERATE INTENSITY (Figure 6.20)

Change tap up to knee up (increased hip range-of-motion, short-lever leg); change arms to shoulder-high lateral raise (mid-range, long-lever arms).

## STEP TOUCH BYPASS: HIGH INTENSITY (Figure 6.21)

Change knee up to front **kick** (long-lever leg); change arms to forward and overhead, reverse "L" position (upper-range, long-lever arms).

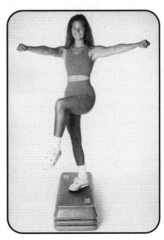

**Figure 6.20** Step Touch Bypass: Moderate intensity.

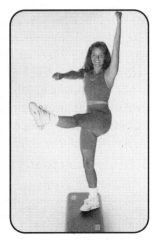

**Figure 6.21** Step Touch Bypass: High intensity.

## SIDE LUNGE: LOW INTENSITY (Figure 6.22)

Perform a **grounded lunge**. From the top of the bench, the body faces forward, foot parallel to bench; arms press down when you step down (low-impact).

## SIDE-LUNGE: MODERATE INTENSITY (Figure 6.23)

Perform a lunge with a small **hop** and 1/4 turn. Opposite arm punches forward. Alternate sides and arms (high-impact).

## SIDE-LUNGE: HIGH INTENSITY (Figure 6.24)

Perform a lunge with a small **propulsion** (a lift with an airborne turn to land in a lunging position) (higher impact).

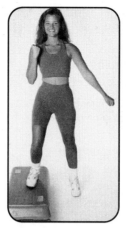
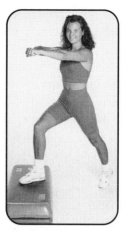
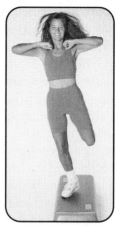

**Figure 6.22** Side Lunge: Low intensity.

**Figure 6.23** Side-Lunge: Moderate intensity.

**Figure 6.24** Side-Lunge: High intensity.

## ■ Double/Multiple Step Training

Movement patterns also can be designed to use two or more step benches. This can add excitement to your step training program by giving your basic steps and step patterns a new twist. This option, called two-stepping or double stepping, incorporates two-step benches per person workout.[11] Participants in two-stepping use the center space between two benches in addition to the outside floor space and tops of both benches to kick, lift, turn, and tap up, down, over, and around the two benches.

Double step is challenging both cardiovascularly and mentally. It is an advanced technique designed for intermediate and advanced participants who are familiar with step terminology, basic steps, and step patterns. Experienced step exercisers, who have developed a high level of skill (both form and technique), endurance, and concentration must also be proficient at following verbal cues because it may not always be possible to see the instructor. Double step training offers the following benefits:

■ It adds variety and helps to combat boredom.

■ Traveling from step to step expends more energy than staying in the same spot.

■ It adds a social element by allowing you to meet new people.

■ It expands movement options.

## Step Placement

Step set-up will vary depending on the number of people in the class. If the class is small, each person may have two steps. The most common placement of the two benches is parallel (Figure 6.25) or at a 90-degree angle (Figure 6.26) — horizontal in front and vertical to the right of you. If the class is large, benches usually are set up in rows

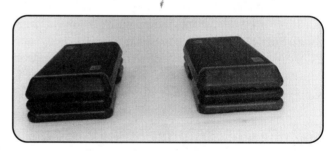

**Figure 6.25** Parallel bench placement.

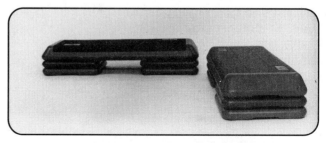

**Figure 6.26** Bench placement: horizontal in front and vertical to your right.

parallel to each other and perpendicular to the front of the room, with an empty bench on the right side at the end of each row. This allows the person at the end of the row to move to the right onto a step bench (Figures 6.27 and 6.28).

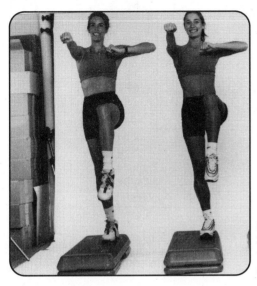

**Figure 6.27**
Step up on the home step.

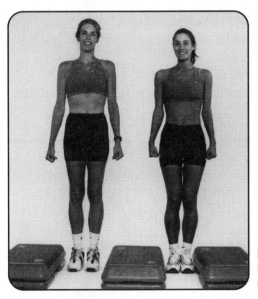

**Figure 6.28**
Exit on the right side.

Prior to class, it is important to set up rows evenly with 14" to 22" between each step. Rows should be staggered to allow participants to view the instructor. In addition, all the benches in the row should be the same height.

## Terminology

In addition to being familiar with step terminology, you need to learn the terms used to identify which step bench you are working on, which side of the bench you are on, and traveling to the other bench. Common terms used in double stepping include:

| | |
|---|---|
| **home:** | the step bench you start on |
| **away or neighbor:** | the step bench you move to |
| **outside:** | outside edge of each step bench |
| **inside:** | area between two step benches; sides of benches closest to each other |
| **double over:** | beginning on the outside edge, go over first the home step bench and then the away step bench (Figures 6.29–6.32) |
| **exit right and stay:** | get off the bench and perform the next step on that bench |
| **transfer or switch:** | go to the other bench, either home or away, depending upon which one you are on now. |

## Double Over (moving left)

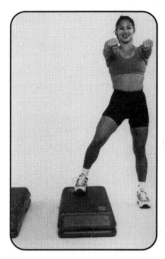
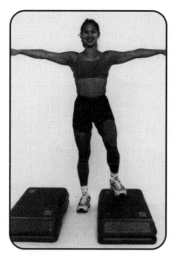
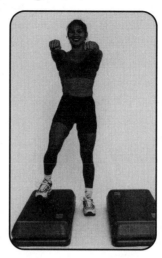
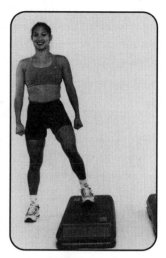

**Figure 6.29**    **Step up L** home step

**Figure 6.30**    **Exit L** home step

**Figure 6.31**    **Step up L** away step

**Figure 6.32**    **Exit L** away step

## Combining Movements

When putting moves together, identifying the number of counts in each of the movements is essential for the flow of the class and the safety and balance of the combinations.

Options for moving from step to step include:

- From the end
- From the outside
  - Double over
  - Straddle transfer
- From the inside
  - Inside turn (Figure 6.33–6.36)
  - V step travel forward (Figure 6.37–6.40)

## Inside Turn

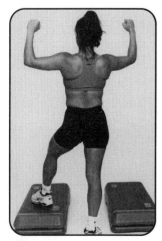
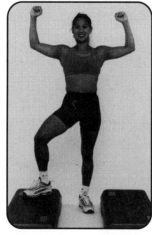
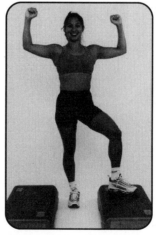
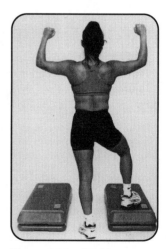

**Figure 6.33**    **"Up"** home step.

**Figure 6.34**    **"Exit"** home step.

**Figure 6.35**    **"Up"** away step.

**Figure 6.36**    **"Exit"** away step.

Turn step on the home step and turn step on the away step

**V-Step Travel Forward**
R

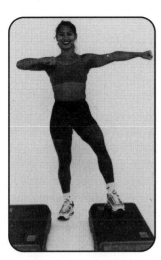 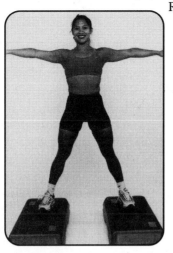 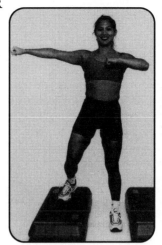 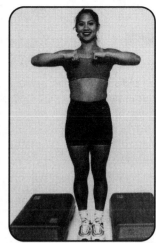

**Figure 6.37**　"Up R."　　**Figure 6.38**　"Up L."　　**Figure 6.39**　"Down" and forward R.　　**Figure 6.40**　"Down" and forward L.

|   | L | R | L |   |   |
|---|---|---|---|---|---|
|   |   | up | up | down & forward | down & forward |

## SUMMARY

Appropriate movement progression is an essential component to ensure safety and for preventing exercise-related injuries. Your aerobic fitness level, skill level, health status, and personal needs or goals determine when you can incorporate variety.

Varying the step training workout offers a number of advantages:

▪ It allows participants with completely different fitness levels and needs to participate in the same class.

▪ By providing many options to accomplish individual program needs, participants are motivated to work within their own fitness and skill levels.

▪ It allows everyone to immediately experience improvement in cardiovascular endurance (the ability to perform more repetitions and work for longer periods), strength development of the musculoskeletal system, and performance improvement of the motor skills involved in step training.

The first advantage described how to increase and decrease intensity (the amount of work you

do, measured as heartbeats per minute). To *increase* intensity, participants safely and progressively work toward ultimately using the maximums presented, unless physical limitations prohibit doing so. To *decrease* intensity, the lesser or minimums in the variables are selected.

The possibilities for step training combinations are endless. Although the basic steps and basic step patterns are simple, combining the steps in various ways can be challenging. Advanced step movements can add excitement and variety to your program. Once you master a complicated combination, you experience a sense of great satisfaction from achieving something that was very complex.

Exercise effectiveness and safety depends mainly on the movements you select and the sequence of those movements (or the way in which you combine them). By adding variety, such as propulsions, traveling and repeater moves, and arm movements, you can vary the intensity to meet your fitness level. Create your own step patterns by using Exercise 6.1, "Creating Your Own Step Training Combinations."

## EXERCISE 6.1

### ■ Creating Your Own Step Training Combinations

*Directions:* Following all of the guidelines you have been given in Chapters 5 and 6, create your own patterns. For safety reasons, only three sides of the bench can be used in a pattern. Start with a bench approach from the end, front, side, top, or diagonal and proceed, incorporating multiple basic step patterns and multiple bench approaches.

1. Indicate the location of the weight-bearing foot (WBF) to start the pattern, freeing the other foot to then be step #1.

2. Begin the pattern by locating a "1" up on the bench (or down on the floor), followed by the location of the next step, identified as "2."

3. Continue locating steps 3–8, then 9–16, identifying any step that has a key directive (e.g., ⑧ is a tap non-weight-bearing move; ⑫ is an astride position).

4. Identify any bypass step movement with a double circle around the non-weight-bearing foot location and labeling the type of bypass move (for example, ⑤ fwd. kick).

5. List arm gestures to accompany each step movement, plus any additional creative building technique pointers (sounds, and so on) below, at right. Enjoy being creative!

## STEPS:

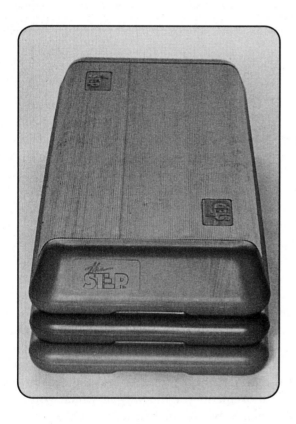

## ARM GESTURES TO STEP #:

1. _____

2. _____

3. _____

4. _____

5. _____

6. _____

7. _____

8. _____

9. _____

10. _____

11. _____

12. _____

13. _____

14. _____

15. _____

16. _____

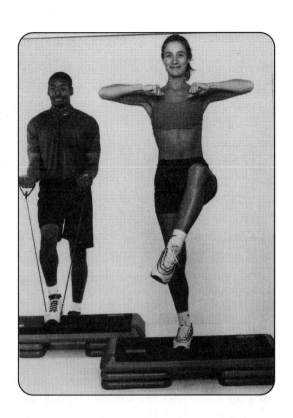

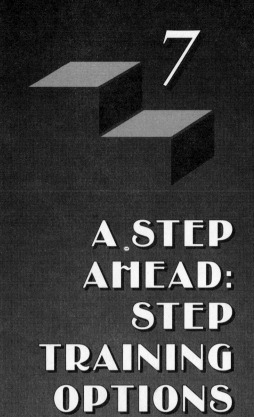

# A STEP AHEAD: STEP TRAINING OPTIONS

**M**any people find it difficult to adhere to an exercise program. Reasons why people fail to exercise include time constraints, lack of results once they start, and boredom. Combining fitness modalities can be a fun way to add variety to your workout. **Combination training** incorporates a variety of activities or modes of training within one class format or workout. The activities and parameters can vary depending on the specific goals to be achieved. Slide, jump rope, high/low impact movements, athletic movements, and calisthenics are all aerobic activities that allow you to customize your workouts. This chapter provides guidelines and suggestions for workout formats, exercise selection, equipment, and efficient training techniques.

## ■■■■ Aerobic Class Format Options

Before exploring different modes of aerobic training (slide, jump rope, sports conditioning, and high/low or combination impact aerobics), consider the different class format options: *continuous*, *circuit*, and *interval*. The most common of these is the *continuous* format, in which the movements and activities selected keep the heart rate within the training heart rate zone throughout the entire cardiovascular/aerobic segment of the class.

## Circuit Training

The term *circuit* means combining a series of fitness activities in one workout and moving from station to station. In circuit training you move from one station to the next with little or no rest in between.[1] The advantage of circuit training is the multiple benefits of:

▌ Improved cardiovascular endurance

▌ Less risk of injury from overuse

▌ A variety of skill levels working together

▌ Versatility of the various options

A circuit may be designed using all aerobic activities. Step aerobics training circuits, however, usually combine step training (to improve aerobic capacity) with weight training exercises (to develop muscular strength and endurance). By alternating the two modalities of exercise, the completed workout can yield the benefits of a total fitness regime.

How the circuit is planned is key to its success. A few guidelines are:

▌ Alternate step aerobic stations with strength training stations (Table 7.1).

▌ Arrange stations so no two consecutive stations exclusively work the same muscle groups.

▌ Maintain an elevated heart rate by moving quickly between stations.

▌ Perform strength training exercises within your training zone heart rate, using light weights, quick repetitions, and *excellent form*. The focus at the strength training stations is to develop muscular endurance through many repetitions rather than to develop power using heavy weights.

▌ Attempt as many of the suggested stepping movements/patterns/sequences or strength training repetitions of a specific exercise as you can in the predetermined time.

▌ To improve, vary the circuits by *increasing* the
 — number of stations
 — planned step movements/number of reps performed, by allotting more time or speeding up the pace
 — number of times the circuit is repeated.

## Interval Training

Interval training is a method of training that alternates periods of high- and low-intensity movements or work and rest intervals. The *work interval* is the period when continuous high intensity activity is performed, and *rest or recovery interval* is the period between work intervals.[2] Unlike other types of aerobic activity that are continuous or steady state, intervals are intermittent. This type of exercise quickly uses up more oxygen than the body can take in while doing the exercise. This, in turn, causes lactic acids (waste products) to accumulate in the muscles, which leads to exhaustion.

The goal of interval training is to push both the aerobic and anaerobic energy systems. This method of training is used most often by athletes but is becoming more popular among fitness enthusiasts because of the added benefit of being able to maximize your time by training more intensely for longer periods (more total work completed in a shorter time), increasing your steady state threshold, increasing your total utilization of fat and increasing your caloric expenditure.[3, 4]

### TABLE 7.1   Cardiovascular/Resistance Training Circuit

| Class Segment | Warm Up | Step Aerobics* | Muscle Conditioning |
|---|---|---|---|
| Time | 7 minutes | 2–3 minutes per movement | 1 minute for each exercise |
| Exercises | | Basic step<br>Alternating knee up<br>Corner to corner kick<br>Turn step<br>Over the top<br>Across the top<br>Alternating hamstring curl<br>Straddle down<br>Lunge side (from the top)<br>Lunge back (from the top) | Bicep curls<br>Tricep kick back<br>Squats<br>Lateral raises<br>Upright row |

*Add variations to the basic steps and basic step patterns

In a step interval training workout, intervals may alternate between step movements using propulsion, such as *run up* (Figures 7.1 and 7.2), and movements that allow the heart rate to come down (basic, v-step, and the like). A cycle (or repetition) consists of a work interval and a recovery interval. When designing an interval training program, the following four variables should be considered:

- Intensity of work
- Recovery interval
- Duration (time) of the work
- Recovery interval.[5]

These variables also depend on the participant's fitness level (see Table 7.2). Your fitness level may be determined by your ability to recover from a work interval. The shorter the recovery interval and the longer the work interval (performed at or above 85% maximum ability), the more challenging the workout.

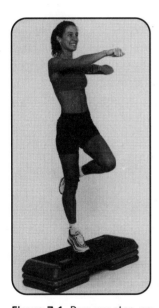

**Figure 7.1** Run up: step up left with propulsion.

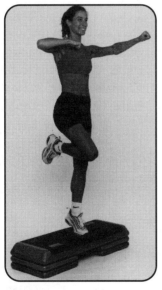

**Figure 7.2** Run up: step up right with propulsion.

## Activities for Circuit or Interval Training

The following exercises are a sample of the activities that can be incorporated into a step training interval or circuit workout.

### Slide Training

Slide training is a high-intensity exercise that uses lateral motion training to achieve cardiovascular and muscular conditioning. This method of training utilizes the adductors and abductors (inner and outer thigh) muscles. Slide training involves moving from side to side across a slick surface.[6] Socks, slippers, or booties are worn over your shoes and allow you to slide across the board.

Like steps, slides (rigid plastic that does not bend or fold and must be hung or stored flat **or** a flexible linoleum-type surface that can be rolled to store) come in various lengths and styles. Slides vary in length from 5 feet to 8 feet. The length you use depends on three variables:

- Your leg length (not height)
- Your fitness level
- Your training goal.

Highly fit and/or long-limbed individuals may prefer a longer board. Shorter and longer boards may both be used to meet the demands of the activity and training goals.[7]

#### BODY POSITIONS

*Front position* (Figure 7.3): Body faces forward with one foot in contact with the end ramp; stance should be comfortable.

*End position* (Figure 7.4): Stand sideways in relation to the slide and face the end ramp; toes are in contact with the end ramp; stance should be comfortable.

*Center position* (Figure 7.5): Body is positioned in the center of the board, facing front.

**TABLE 7.2    Interval Training Variables**

|  | Beginner | Intermediate | Advanced |
|---|---|---|---|
| Intensity of Work Interval | 70%–75% | 75%–85% | 85%–95% |
| Intensity of Recovery Interval | 30%–35% | 35%–40% | 40%–45% |
| Duration (Time) Work Interval | 60–90 seconds | 90 seconds | 90–105 seconds |
| Duration (Time) Recovery Interval | 3–4 minutes | 3 minutes | 2–3 minutes |

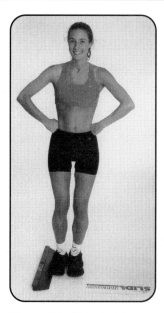

**Figure 7.3** Slide training — front position.

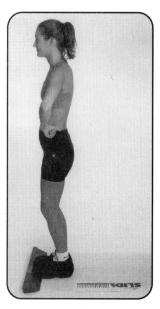

**Figure 7.4** Slide training — end position.

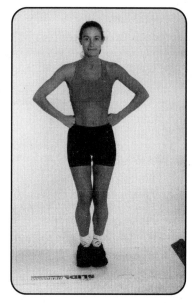

**Figure 7.5** Slide training — center position.

## STANCES

*Upright stance*: Used for basic slide, torso is erect and knees maintain a slight bend; hands may be placed on the hips or upper thighs to maintain balance and distribute weight evenly, or behind your back; shoulders are aligned over the hips.

*Athletic ready stance* (Figure 7.6): Used for low-profile slide; bend in the hips and knees is deeper than in the upright stance. Place hands on the front of the thighs, well above the knees. When you need less support and stability, place your hands behind your back.

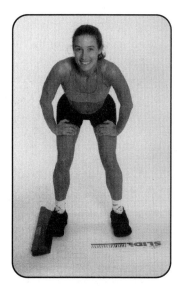

**Figure 7.6** Slide training — athletic ready stance.

## HOW TO SLIDE[8]

1. Before stepping onto the slide surface, place slide socks over your shoes.
2. Center your weight and carefully get a feel for the slick surface of the slide.
3. Standing on one end, flex your knees, push off the bumper, and glide to the other side.
4. Keep both feet flat on the slide surface. For all movements, knees should always be in alignment with the feet and toes.
5. Concentrate on maintaining your posture — upper body aligned, rib cage lifted, abdominals tight.
6. Gradually increase the force with which your trail leg pushes off from the bumper, and get used to allowing the opposite leg (lead leg) to absorb the impact of contacting the bumper.
7. When you are comfortable with the sliding motion, add arm movements.
8. Keep the upper body relaxed, supported, and steady at all times.
9. When you are ready, experiment with various arm movements and sliding at different tempos.

## SLIDE MOVEMENT

In slide training, the *basic slide*, or side-to-side movement, can be broken down into three phases:

1. *Push-off* (Figure 7.7): A strong trail-leg push propels the body across the slide.

2. *Glide phase* The body moves across the slide.

3. *Contact and recovery phase* (Figure 7.8): As the lead leg contacts the other end of the ramp, the trail leg helps slow you down, stabilize, and stop the movement.

## BASIC MOVES

*Fencing Slide* (Figure 7.9): Begin in the upright stance, **rotate lead leg outward** from the hip, and cut through the center of the slide as though you are fencing. Keep knee in line with hips then reverse directions.

    *Reverse Fencing Slide* (Figure 7.10): **Rotate trail leg outward** so it cuts through the center of the board.

### Slide Touches/Bypass Moves

■ *Front slide touch:* Once the lead leg reaches the end of the slide, lift the trail leg in front of leading leg. Keep hips square.

■ *Rear slide touch:* Bring trail leg back behind lead leg. Wait until you make solid contact with ramp before you initiate the touch.

■ *Slide knee lift:*

**Front** (Figure 7.11): Complete basic slide, then lift knee of trail leg straight up.

Cross-knee lift: Rotate hips and cross knee in front.

Side: Rotate trail leg outward and lift knee.

■ *Hamstring curl:* Complete slide and lift heel to seat using controlled movement.

■ *Slide leg lift:* Once you have made contact with end:

Side leg lift (Figure 7.12)

Kick forward (Figure 7.13)

Rear leg lift: Use athletic stance and lift leg to the back.

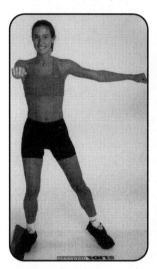

**Figure 7.7** Slide movement — push-off.

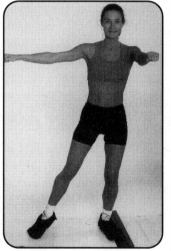

**Figure 7.8** Slide movement — contact and recovery phase.

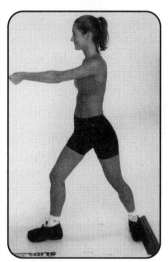

**Figure 7.9** Fencing slide.

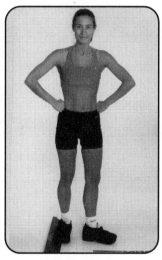

**Figure 7.10** Reverse fencing slide.

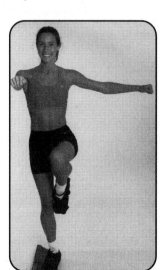

**Figure 7.11** Slide knee lift.

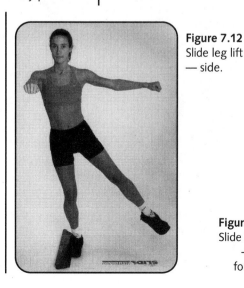

**Figure 7.12** Slide leg lift — side.

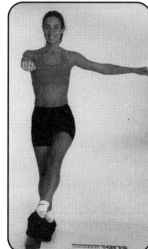

**Figure 7.13** Slide leg lift — kick forward.

## SLIDE VARIATIONS

▌ *Slide lunge*

Side lunge: Lunge side with trail leg; bring leg back to end before initiating.

Basic slide movement: Maintain contact with end of ramp.

Rear lunge: Face end of the ramp and lunge back (similar to repeaters).

Depth of lunge will determine intensity.

▌ *Cross-country ski* (Figure 7.14): From the end with toes touching and perpendicular to the ramp.

Narrow: small range of motion

Wide: large range of motion

▌ *Slide squat* (Figure 7.15): Slide in the upright stance, and squat after you make contact with the end of the ramp.

▌ *Slide lift* (Figure 7.16): As you complete the basic slide, rise onto your toes as you lift your knee; do not hop.

▌ *Squat pull* (Figure 7.17): Start in center position and use your inner/outer thigh muscles to slide legs out; drop into a squat with feet slightly wider than shoulder-width apart, then pull legs in. This movement resembles a jumping jack but the entire foot remains in contact with the slide.

▌ *Wide slide:* Bring in trail leg slightly.

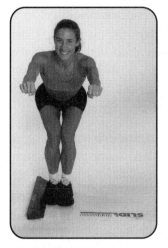

**Figure 7.15** Slide squat.

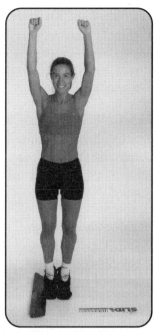

**Figure 7.16** Slide lift.

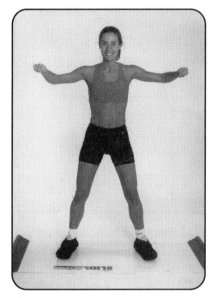

**Figure 7.17** Slide squat pull.

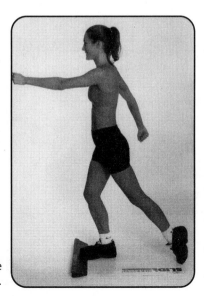

**Figure 7.14** Slide cross-country ski.

## Jump Rope

Jumping rope is a strenuous activity that uses approximately three times more energy than leisure walking. This high-impact activity is not suited for everyone. Inactive individuals and those with joint and back problems should not participate in this form of aerobic exercise. Others with exercise experience should have no problem.

A "giving" surface upon which to jump is preferable. The rope should reach your armpits when held down tightly under your feet, with a few extra inches, or a handle, with which to hold the rope comfortably (Figure 7.18). If the rope has no handles, tape the ends or tie knots at the ends to prevent fraying.

Among the variety of jump ropes on the market are beaded, licorice, leather, and cotton ropes. Beaded ropes and leather ropes are the best choice. Licorice (plastic) ropes get tangled more frequently, and cotton ropes are rather difficult to use because they are so lightweight.

The following procedure is recommended for jumping rope:

1. When you warm up, be sure to static-stretch all the muscles of the leg, with special attention to the calf, heel cord, and shin areas.

2. Begin the aerobic segment with 6 minutes, progressing to a 20-minute workout. Jump low with "soft" knees for efficiency, and only high enough to clear the rope (less than 1 inch).

3. Use the wrists, not shoulders, to turn the rope. Keep your arms bent and close to the body at hip-to-waist level with palms facing slightly upward and forward.

4. Restrict continuous jumping to 1-minute intervals at 120–140 revolutions per minute, a moderate pace. Alternate 1-minute segments with non-jumping, low-impact aerobics such as marching or power walking. Music should range from 120–140 beats per minute, to assist in timing and rhythm.

5. Use rate of perceived exertion to monitor your intensity because it will allow you a minute-to-minute monitoring of how you feel.

6. Provide a 5–10 minute cool-down, including non-jumping, low-impact moves, and flexibility and relaxation for 5 minutes, static stretching again for the leg muscles used.[9]

Jump rope exercises illustrated are the

- *Two-foot jump* (Figure 7.19)
- *Boxer shuffle* (Figure 7.20): Shift your weight slightly from left to right.

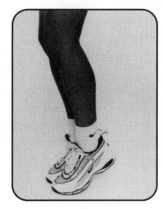

**Figure 7.19** Jump rope — two-foot jump.

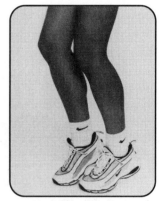

**Figure 7.20** Jump rope — boxer shuffle.

- *Leg kicks* (Figure 7.21): Alternate right and left kicks in front of you.
- *Cross-country ski* (Figure 7.22): Alternate right and left foot forward and backward.

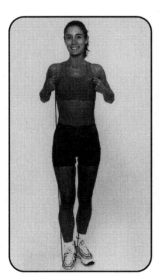

**Figure 7.18** Determining proper length of jump rope.

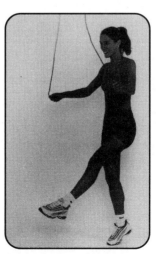

**Figure 7.21** Jump rope — leg kicks.

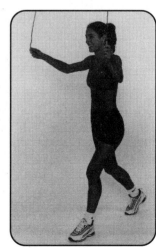

**Figure 7.22** Jump rope — cross-country ski.

■ *Criss-cross/jack* (Figure 7.23): Cross the rope in front; jump and cross legs; jump and land wide-stride.

■ *Leg curl* (Figure 7.24): Alternate lifting right and left heel to seat.

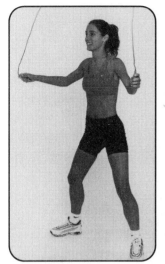
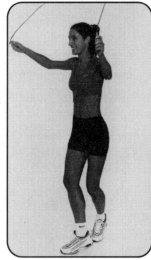

**Figure 7.23** Jump rope — criss-cross.

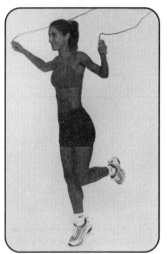

**Figure 7.24** Jump rope — leg curl.

## Sports Conditioning

A sports conditioning workout uses calisthenics (push-ups, sit-ups, jumping-jacks, and the like) and movements that simulate sports like box aerobics and sport sprints. Movement patterns are basic and simple to follow, emphasizing coordination, speed, agility, and quickness. These fun movements can be a great way to energize your workout.

### BOX AEROBICS

*Box aerobics* is a popular form of aerobic training that utilizes the upper body during the aerobic segment of the workout. Researchers have found that an hour of non contact boxing uses as much energy as running 5⅝ miles in an hour.[10]

A box aerobic class incorporates the "boxer shuffle" (shifting your weight in little bounces from left to right) while throwing punches and kicking. Before throwing a punch, you must have the proper stance: feet a comfortable distance apart, both knees slightly bent, arms close to the side and slightly to the front of the body (Figure 7.25). Punching movements used in boxing include jabs (Figure 7.26), extending the arm without locking out the elbow, and leading with the first two knuckles; upper cuts (Figure 7.27), swinging your arm up and following with the elbow; and hooks (Figure 7.28), using the back muscles to

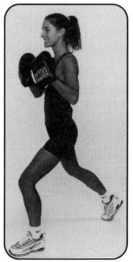
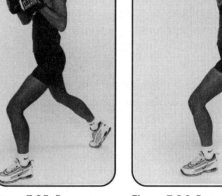

**Figure 7.25** Box aerobics — stance.

**Figure 7.26** Box aerobics — jabs.

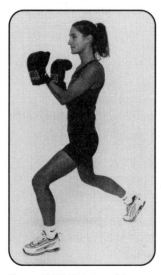
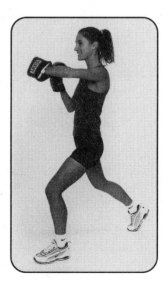

**Figure 7.27** Box aerobics — upper cuts.

**Figure 7.28** Box aerobics — hooks.

propel your arm across your chest.[11] Kicks also may be added to a box aerobic workout (Figure 7.29).

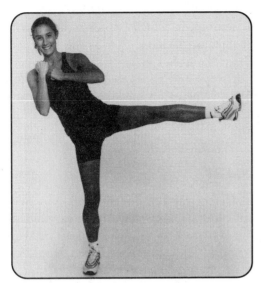

**Figure 7.29** Box aerobics — kicks.

## COMBINING SPORTS MOVEMENTS

Many athletes and fitness enthusiasts select sports conditioning as a way to enhance athletic performance. Sport movements (Table 7.3) can be combined

**TABLE 7.3    Sports Conditioning Movements**

| Calisthenics | Boxing | Sport Sprints |
|---|---|---|
| jacks | ready stance | tennis |
| shuffle (Figure 7.30) | duck & weave | football |
| squat | punches | baseball |
| fast feet | jab | basketball |
| jumps | uppercut | volleyball |
| slides | hook | |
| | kicks — | |
| |    front, side, back | |

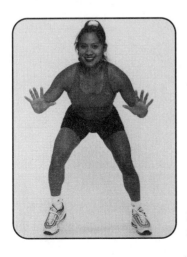

**Figure 7.30** Sports movements — shuffle.

for a station-to-station circuit workout, unison circuit (all participants performing the same activity), or interval workout (alternating between high and low intensity).

Other Options include:

- Pyramid jumps/graduated steps
- Court or obstacle course (Figure 7.31)
- Relay, sport sprints.

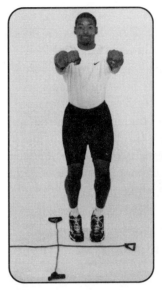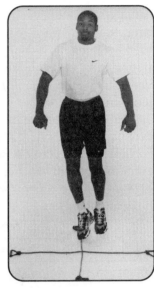

**Figure 7.31** a. Obstacle course station. b. Hop over the tube.

## Combination High-/Low-Impact Aerobics (CIA or Combo-Impact)

The combination style of movement utilizes characteristics of both high- and low-impact movement, which can be a safe and exciting blend. Combination high/low-impact choreography can be defined in two ways.[12]

1. *Routines that offer both a high-impact and a low-impact version of a movement.* Programs that offer both of these work best in classes with mixed fitness levels so individual participants can select the amount of impact appropriate for them. A beginner in the program, therefore, may choose to do the low-impact version, whereas an experienced dance-exerciser may be more challenged by the high-impact movements.

2. *Routines combining a series of varied high-impact and a series of varied low-impact movements.*

This style lends itself well to classes of experienced aerobics exercisers whose primary concern is to improve cardiorespiratory fitness while minimizing the risk of injury.

Combination-impact aerobics offers a wide range of choices and possibilities. It allows you to individualize how much physical stress you choose to experience safely at various times and stages of your life according to your fitness level, personal goals, and special interests. Especially if you are a beginner, coming off an illness or injury, obese, older, or pregnant, you will want to choose the less biomechanically stressful, low-impact movements. Athletes in training and well-conditioned, injury-free individuals may choose the high-impact movements and series more frequently, or even exclusively.

The unique feature of a combination approach is that participants can choose (from the various possibilities) the impact that best fits their current needs. Some people, of course, cannot participate in the high-impact movements at all because of permanent physical limitations.

## Choosing a Format

When determining which format to use, you should consider effectiveness and efficiency. Because of the limited time a person usually has to work out, time efficiency should be a major goal. Identify your equipment needs in advance, and have everything available before starting your workout. Three options are:

1. *Alternate activities* and then repeat them in the same order (for example: step, jump rope, muscle conditioning, repeat sequence).

2. *Linear progression* in which you move from one activity to the next without repeating activities.

3. *Simultaneous alternating activity* (for use in a class setting), in which two or more activities are performed at the same time as the students rotate between them. For example, with a limited number of steps and slides, half the group may perform movements on the step while the other half performs movements on the slide, and then the groups switch.

## SUMMARY

During a step training interval or circuit workout, different modes of training can be combined when selecting activities to perform during the work and rest intervals. The activities selected should complement one another by working opposing muscle groups when doing resistance exercises or vary the musculoskeletal stress, such as step (knee flexion) and slide (hip abduction and adduction). Among the nearly limitless combinations possible are:

▌ slide training

▌ step and high/low impact (combination) aerobics

▌ step and jump rope

▌ step and sports conditioning

Combination training adds excitement, and relieves boredom, helping you to stay motivated and adhere to your exercise program.

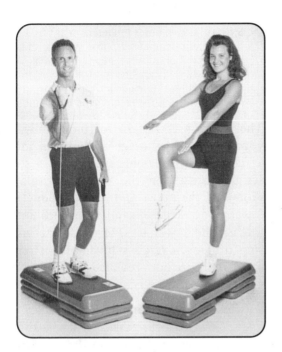

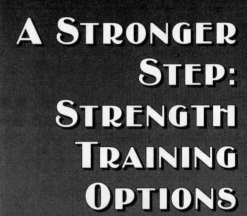

# A STRONGER STEP: STRENGTH TRAINING OPTIONS

Options for using the step/bench are unlimited. It can be used not only for aerobic conditioning (as has been presented so far) but also during the anaerobic phase of the workout for improving muscle strength and endurance through strength training (Figures 8.1 and 8.2). To complement the cardiovascular step portion of the workout, include progressive resistance training techniques *using the step/bench in conjunction with a variety of equipment* such as hand-held light weights, elastic tubing, and bands.

## ▊ Benefits of Step/Bench with Strength

Benefits to be attained by adding a progressive resistance strength training component to the step aerobics workout are:[1]

▊ Develop stronger muscles to help with the tasks of daily living;

▊ Improve resiliency (elasticity)

▊ Restore and maintain muscle balance, to prevent injuries

▊ Improve body composition (greater lean, less fat tissue)

▊ Increase firmness and tone of muscles (greater bulk and definition)

▊ Overall well-being and functional efficiency (feel better and move easier).

When combined with other strength training equipment, the bench/step can be an innovative piece of exercise equipment.

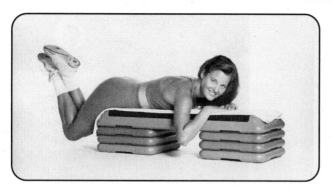

**Figure 8.1** Step bench with strength. Use step bench to allow full range of motion.

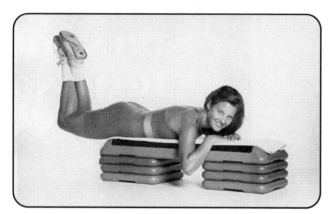

**Figure 8.2** Step bench with strength. Use step bench to support the body.

Three advantages in using it when performing strength training exercises are[2] that it:

- Provides support for the pelvis, low back, and neck, which increases effectiveness and decreases the chance of injury.
- Affords the opportunity to work with or against weight resistance by letting gravity work for or against you.
- Increases the range-of-motion possible for each exercise, allowing greater muscular contraction. (Because of the elevation of the step, you can extend the movements and get a "pre-stretch" for full range-of-motion.)

## ■ Prescription for Strength Training Exercises

The strength training segment is optional in the step aerobics class setting. Because it is a vital component of total physical fitness, however, most step aerobics classes today include 10–20 minutes of strength-training to provide a well-balanced and complete

fitness program. Guidelines from the American College of Sports Medicine state:

> Strength training of a moderate intensity, sufficient to develop and maintain fat-free weight, should be an integral part of an adult fitness program. One set of eight to twelve repetitions of eight to ten exercises that condition the major muscle groups, at least two days per week, is the recommended minimum.[3]

The above prescription for more fully developing your lean (fat-free) weight is shown in Table 8.1.

The strength training segment in a step aerobics setting focuses on the following isolated muscle groups of the upper and middle body. (Because the lower body, which includes the hips and buttocks, thighs, and lower legs, is used extensively during step training, exercises to develop strength in the lower body are not presented in this text.) They are:

- Upper body: chest, upper back, shoulders, arms
- Midsection: abdominals, lower back.

Exercises presented here use the following types of weight-resistance modes:

- Commercial rubber resistance bands
- Commercial rubber resistance tubing alone, or with the aid of the bench
- Gravity-assisted techniques, in which the bench is placed in an incline or decline position, with 1–4 pound hand-held weights, resistance tubing, or using your own body weight as the sole resistance.

Note: The bench is **not** designed for using free weights that weigh 10 pounds or more.[4]

The exercises illustrated and described here have been categorized according to location of the muscle group(s) benefited (upper body/mid-section) using a variety of equipment. Figure 8.3 illustrates the major muscle groups[5] to be strength-trained. Table 8.2 identifies the exercises that will accomplish the training.

**TABLE 8.1   Prescription for Strength Training**

| Set | Reps | Varieties of Exercises | Minimum Days/Week |
|-----|------|------------------------|-------------------|
| 1 | 8–12 | 8–10 targeting major muscle groups | 2 (with max.: 4/week, or every other day) |

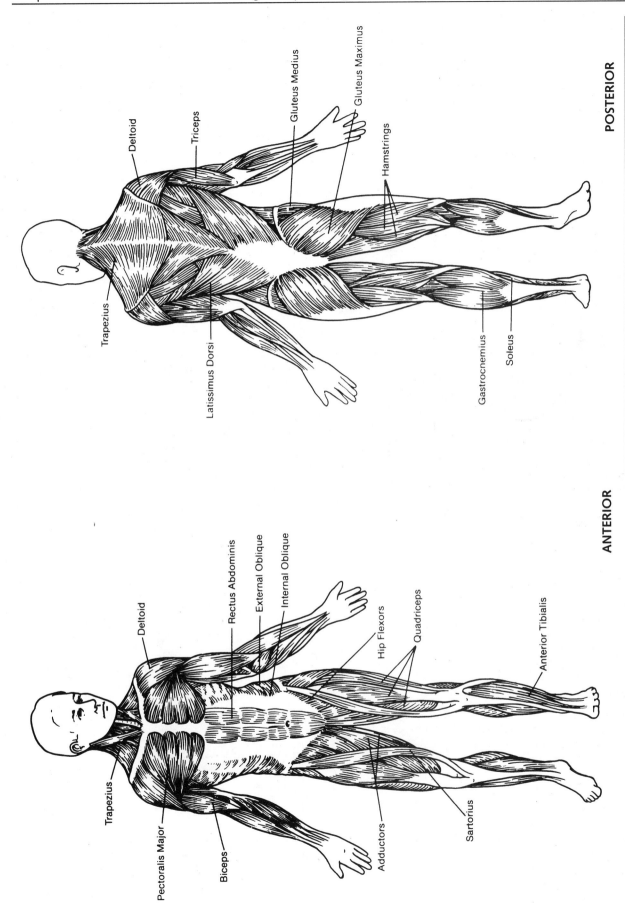

**POSTERIOR**

Deltoid

Triceps

Gluteus Medius

Gluteus Maximus

Hamstrings

Trapezius

Latissimus Dorsi

Gastrocnemius

Soleus

**ANTERIOR**

Deltoid

Rectus Abdominis

External Oblique

Internal Oblique

Hip Flexors

Quadriceps

Anterior Tibialis

Trapezius

Pectoralis Major

Biceps

Adductors

Sartorius

Source: *Weight Training for Life*, by James L. Hesson (Morton Publishing, 1985).

**Figure 8.3** Major muscles to be strength-trained.

**TABLE 8.2  Strength Training Exercises Using Various Forms of Resistance with Step/Bench**

| UPPER BODY<br>Chest/Upper Back/Shoulders/Arms<br>(Figures 8.6–8.24) | MID-SECTION<br>Abdominals/Low Back<br>(Figures 8.25–8.27) |
| --- | --- |
| Chest press | Gravity-assisted curl-up with weights |
| Bent-arm chest cross-over | Reverse curl-up |
| Chest fly | Back extension |
| Straight-arm side-raise | |
| Overhead press | |
| Overhead triceps extension | |
| Deltoid raise with bent knees | |
| Upright row with bent knees | |
| Triceps kick (press) back with bent knees | |
| Biceps curl with bent knees | |

> *For comfort and safety, place a towel on the bench platform when lying on it.*

## Variety of Resistance

To incorporate variety into your program, consider the following forms of resistance:

1. *Your own body (or parts)* lifted and lowered[6] against gravity as the weight resistance, as in push-ups and curl-ups (see Figures 4.17 and 4.21) in Chapter 4. To progressively increase the resistance involved in lifting your body's weight against gravity, a strategically placed free-weight is used (on the sternum for a curl-up, Figure 8.25, or between the shoulder blades for a push-up, for example).

2. *Hand-held weights* (not wrist-weights) in controlled movement or placed on the body in the key locations to add weight resistance to the body part being lifted and lowered.

3. *Rubber resistance bands*, 9", 12", or 16" long, in widths of ¼–1½ inches. The length and width are selected according to whether the exercise is for upper or lower body, and for your current strength fitness level in the muscle group being trained.

4. *Rubber resistance tubing*, approximately 3–4½ feet long so you can adjust it according to your height in a range of light to heavy thickness that you select according to your current level of strength fitness.

5. A combination of *all the above*, using a step-bench in a level position, or in the gravity-assisted incline or decline positions. You will begin to realize,

from the exercises shown, that the possibilities for variety in the strength training segment are fun, exciting, inexpensive, and unlimited.

Options 3, 4, and 5 are shown in Figure 8.4. The principles for using these unique pieces of equipment are discussed next.

## Using Resistance Bands and Tubing

Instructions for using either resistance bands or tubing are as follows.

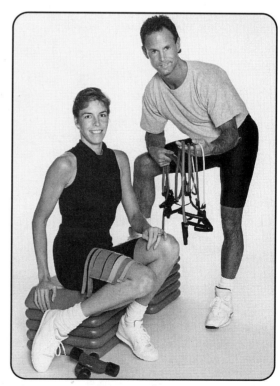

**Figure 8.4** Various equipment to use for resistance when exercising.

- Select bands and tubing based on your fitness level.

- Always inspect the bands and tubing before each use, for nicks and tears resulting from continued use.

- Never, under any circumstances, tie pieces of band and tubing together.

- Always exhibit proper body alignment and good posture while exercising.

- To assure safety, keep your face turned slightly away from the direction of movement.

- While performing single-limb, upper-body movements, always anchor the band between one hand and the thigh, hip, side, or shoulder, depending on the movement.

- Always anchor the tubing under the ball of one foot, or both feet (when not using it with the bench), depending on your level of fitness and the desired amount of tension you wish to create.

- Always control the bands and tubing, especially during the return phase of the movement. Do not let them control you.

- Perform 8 to 10 repetitions of each exercise. When using one arm or leg, switch sides so the same muscle group is worked an equal number of repetitions on both sides of the body. Be sure to work all muscle groups with equal intensity and repetitions at each session, to avoid muscular imbalance.[7]

### BANDS

Bands are available in a variety of sizes, allowing you to vary the intensity of your workout.[8] Suggested sizes:

- Beginner
  ⅜" upper body (pink or light blue)
  ⅜" or ⅝" lower body

- Intermediate
  ⅝" upper body (light blue)
  ⅝" lower body

- Advanced
  ¾" upper body (dark blue)
  ¾" lower body

### TUBING

Tubing (see Figure 8.5) is available in a variety of sizes to vary the intensity of your workout.[9]

- Beginner
  Very light and light tubing (yellow or green)

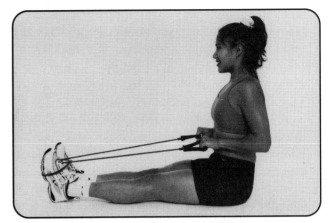

**Figure 8.5** Seated lower leg flexor and extensor — using rubber tubing.

- Intermediate
  Light and medium tubing (green or red)
- Advanced
  Heavy tubing (blue)

## ■ Principles of Strength Training

If possible, plan approximately 10–20 minutes for strength training during your workout, applying the following principles:

- Precede and follow muscle strengthening exercises by stretching exercises specific to the muscles that are made to work against resistance. Any muscle group strengthened by exercise also should be stretched regularly to prevent abnormal contraction of resting length.[10]

- Of key importance, stabilize your joints and your spine before beginning each exercise.

- Perform each movement using a smooth, continuous, full range-of-motion action for the joint/muscle group involved, and keep the timing of the movement (usually slow) totally under your control. Ballistic (rapid or jerky) movements increase the risk of injury.

- For proper timing, take approximately 2 seconds to perform the overcoming-resistance-action (concentric) phase, and from 2 to 4 seconds (at least the same time, or up to twice as long) during the release or lowering (eccentric) phase to return to the starting position of each exercise.[11]

- Exhale during the lifting, overcoming resistance-action move; inhale during the release or lowering and return. (Exception: During overhead pressing movements, inhale as you lift).[12]

- Use visualization and self-talk here. Plan concentrated thoughts to accompany your lifting/exhale and lowering/inhale movements.

- Design the repetitions of each exercise and the sets of repetitions according to the progressive resistance format. Begin with one to three sets of 8–12 repetitions for most exercises. (Exception: For abdominal work, begin your program by performing two sets of 15–30 repetitions per set). Select 8–10 exercises that condition the major muscle groups of your body for at least two of your aerobic sessions per week, if you have no other separate strength training program.

- When you become jerky, are not smooth, continuous, and rhythmical in the move, and are not using the full range-of-motion possible around your joints, you've completed your lower limit possible for that set. Make a record of this number. This lower limit becomes the baseline to which you attempt to add more repetitions as soon as possible.

- Do not continue to add more repetitions without adding resistance. Adding resistance in increasingly greater increments (say, from 1 to 4 pounds if using hand weights, or thicker rubber if using bands/tubing) will provide the added resistance you need over the course of your program.

- Perform strength training on isolated muscle groups on an every-other-day basis. Your muscles need a day to recover, so don't incorporate a program to strength train with resistance (weights/bands/tubing) daily. An alternative to this program is to perform strength training exercises with resistance (weights/bands/tubing) for the *upper half of your body one day*, and for the *lower half of your body the next day*. You thus are alternating the days the muscles are strength training.

- Allow brief rest periods between bouts of vigorous exercises. This is the most efficient way to improve strength. (The timeframe for rest is defined as regaining a normal breathing pattern.)

### ▬ Bench and Tubing Exercises

Incline and decline, adhere to the following advice.[13]

- Be sure bench blocks are locked into place.
- Make sure there is no more than two blocks' difference from one end to other.
- Place a mat or towel on top of the bench platform.

- To sit on the bench, place your pelvis in the middle of the bench platform, then adjust your hips.
- Use your hands to push your torso up when in the decline position.
- Avoid the decline position for prolonged periods.
- Maintain tension in the tubing by securing it under key parts of the bench and wrapping extra tubing length in your palm.

### Chest Press (Figures 8.6 and 8.7)

This is an excellent beginning exercise to develop pectoral strength.

**Position** (Figure 8.6): Loop tubing under the step/bench so an end is accessible on both sides. Sit facing outward on the end of the step. Grab a handle in each hand, taking up slack by wrapping the tubing around your hands. Bring your hands shoulder-high, elbows near sides.

**Action** (Figure 8.7): Exhale and press away, shoulder-high, straight out in front of you. Inhale and return.

**Bench and tubing**
**(Pectoralis Major, Anterior Deltoid, Triceps)**

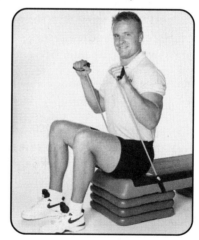

**Figure 8.6** Chest press — position.

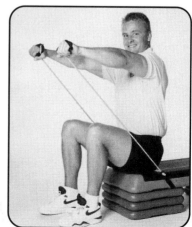

**Figure 8.7** Chest press — action.

## Bent-Arm Chest Cross-Over (Figures 8.8, 8.9)

Adjust bench so two blocks are at the low end and four blocks are at the high end.

**Position** (Figure 8.8): Sit center; move buttocks to lower third of bench; lie with head resting at top. Grasp the tubing that is placed under platform center, near shoulders. Place your feet flat on the floor, with knees in open position, with arms wide open at shoulder level, elbows bent.

**Action** (Figure 8.9): Take cross-punch arm position over chest while pressing your back firmly against the bench, and a "big-hug" position.

### Incline bench and tubing (Pectorals)

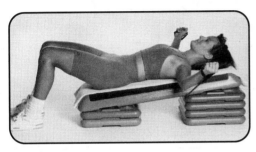

**Figure 8.8**
Bent-arm chest cross-over — position.

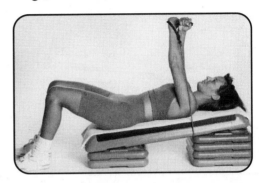

**Figure 8.9**
Bent-arm chest cross-over — action.

## Chest Fly (Figures 8.10, 8.11)

**Position** (Figure 8.10): Lie on your back with buttocks on low end of bench, knees in open position. Hold one hand-weight in each hand above the shoulders, with the arms slightly bent, and wide open.

**Action** (Figure 8.11): Raise weights toward each other directly above you.

### Incline bench and 1–4 pound hand-held weights (Pectorals)

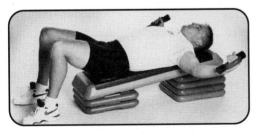

**Figure 8.10**
Chest fly — position.

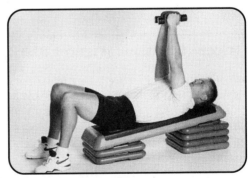

**Figure 8.11**
Chest fly — action.

*The step/bench is adjustable. For all strength training exercises using an incline/decline bench (four block risers at one end, two block risers at the other end), you'll get a fuller range-of-motion as you go through each exercise, allowing greater muscular contraction.*

## Straight-Arm Side Raise (Figures 8.12, 8.13)

**Position** (Figure 8.12): Place tubing in the top notch, between platform and first block, at the low end of bench, giving a little tug to be sure it is secure. Roll up tubing, holding onto the handles, thumbs facing in toward bench.

**Action** (Figure 8.13): Gently lift up until the thumbs face up and above the head. Hold. Lower back to floor.

### Incline bench and tubing (Deltoids)

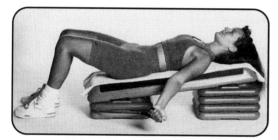

**Figure 8.12**  Straight-arm side raise — position.

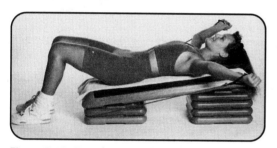

**Figure 8.13**  Straight-arm side raise — action.

## Overhead Press (Figures 8.14, 8.15)

**Position** (Figure 8.14): Prone, with tubing in back of first block's groove, hands starting at sides, wide, and chin resting on incline bench top.

**Action** (Figure 8.15): Press up and forward, ending with thumbs rotating in, and facing each other.

### Incline bench and tubing (Deltoids/Triceps)

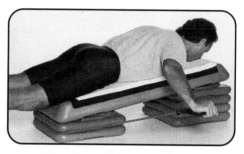

**Figure 8.14**  Overhead press — position.

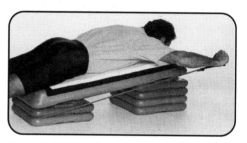

**Figure 8.15**  Overhead press — action

## Overhead Triceps Extension (Figures 8.16, 8.17)

**Position** (Figure 8.16): Place tubing under center of bench so it is next to top blocks and at shoulder height. Raise arms so elbows are in the air and actually pinch in toward each other. The thumbs will start facing the ground.

**Action** (Figure 8.17): Extend up and rotate the palms up toward the ceiling. Thumbs will come up so they face each other. Relax back down. Cue yourself: "Up, press, contract."

### Incline bench and tubing (Triceps)

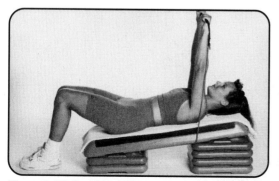

**Figure 8.16**  Overhead Triceps Extension — position.

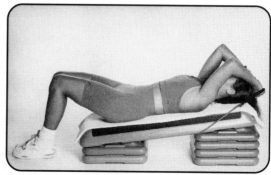

**Figure 8.17**  Overhead Triceps Extension — action.

## Deltoid Raise with Bent Knees (Figure 8.18)

**Position:** Stand on top of bench, feet slightly apart with tubing under center, having fists top/thumbs-in-and-down position.

**Action:** Press up, bending knees, with elbows bent and hands leading, going only to shoulder level or lower. If fatigued, raise arms just halfway, or use lighter tubing.

### Bench and tubing (Deltoids/Trapezius)

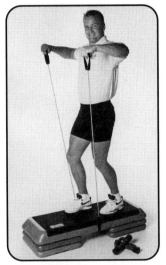

*Bent knees in all of these illustrations assist in keeping a target heart rate, so these exercises can also serve as 1-minute strength training intervals in an aerobic step training with strength intervals program.*

**Figure 8.18** Deltoid Raise with Bent Knees.

## Upright Row (Figures 8.19, 8.20)

**Position** (Figure 8.19): Stand on bench's center/back, feet together, with tubing under center, hands/fists now facing thighs.

**Action** (Figure 8.20): Raise handles up to chin, flaring elbows slightly, shoulder high, keeping spine firmly erect. Bend knees on action.

### Bench and tubing (Deltoids/Trapezius)

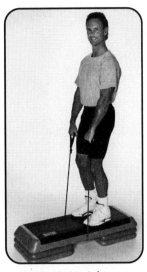

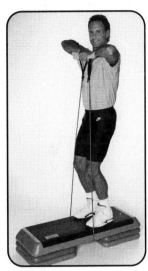

**Figure 8.19** Upright row — position.

**Figure 8.20** Upright row — action.

## Triceps Kick (Press) Back with Bent Knees (Figures 8.21, 8.22)

**Position** (Figure 8.21): Stand on the back third of bench with tubing under center/back. Palms start at sides on thighs, thumbs up.

**Action** (Figure 8.22): Rotate palms out and back to extension, thumbs down. Bend knees on the action.

### Bench and tubing (Triceps)

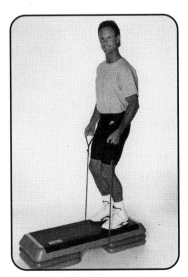

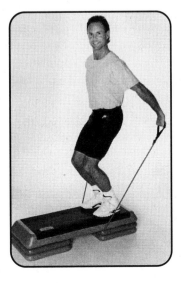

**Figure 8.21** Triceps kick (press) back with bent knees — position.

**Figure 8.22** Triceps kick (press) back with bent knees — action.

## Biceps Curl with Bent Knees (Figures 8.23, 8.24)

**Position** (Figure 8.23): Stand on the back third of bench with tubing under center/back. Hand/fist position now faces thighs.

**Action** (Figure 8.24): Curl up to sky, rotating palms on the way up so they face shoulders. Reverse the rotation for return. Again, bend knees on the action to increase heart rate.

### Bench and tubing (Biceps/Brachialis)

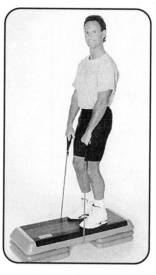 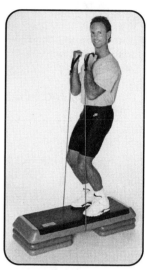

Figure 8.23 Biceps curl with bent knees — position.

**Figure 8.24** Biceps curl with bent knees — action.

## Gravity-Assisted Curl-Up (Figure 8.25)

### Incline bench and 1–4 pound weights (Abdominals)

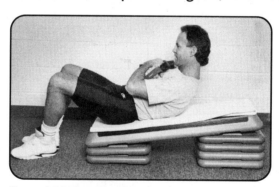

**Figure 8.25** Gravity-assisted curl-up.

Repetitions for abdominal work can be 15–30, and two sets — one before a step aerobics session and one after, because the type of muscle tissue located here responds well to more repetitions for "definition" than other groups of the body. These exercises are to help strengthen sensitive lower back; the low back is completely supported during the abdominal contraction. No "daylight" shows between the bench mat (or towel) on the bench and your shirt in low-back area.

> **Position:** With bench in incline position, straddle and sit on the lower third. Place 1–4 pound freeweights* on sternum (breastbone), with knees flared out wide and heels together, flat on floor. (This leg position works the abdominals and decreases the chance that the hip flexors will help in the movement.)
>
> **Action:** Keeping the lower back on the bench at all times, curl-up, head looking forward. Hold, and contract with your mind thinking ("squ-e-e-e-ze"). This is all the farther you go. Release and curl back down to lying position.

*Adding more weight resistance is optional, but if you do, this is where it should be done. When using weights while on bench, maximum weight is 10 pounds.

## Reverse Curl-Up (Figure 8.26)

Position: Place bench in a decline position. Lie on bench, face up with head at lower end of bench. Grasp lip of platform and top block over your head. Legs are skyward, with hips, knees, and ankles softly bent.

Action: Contract abdominals and raise buttocks, keeping lower back on the platform. Lower.

### Decline bench (Abdominals)

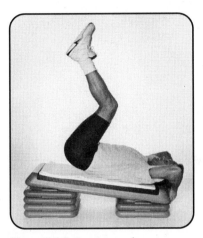

**Figure 8.26** Reverse curl-up.

## Back Extension (Figure 8.27)

Position: Lie prone, with hips on lower third, legs extending off bench, supported by toes on floor. With chin on bench, place hands at hips area.

Action: Contract low back and raise upper chest. Hands may move in a sliding motion backward. Lower.

### Incline bench (Erector Spinae)

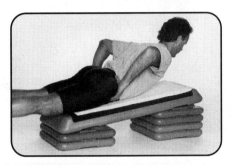

**Figure 8.27** Back extension.

*Remember to breathe evenly during all strength training exercises. To hold your breath and turn red is never acceptable, as your working muscles constantly need oxygen.*

## Combination Upper and Lower Body Exercises (Figures 8.28–8.34)

Upper and lower body exercises may be combined for a complete strength training workout. The following exercises can be performed during the strength training/muscle conditioning segment of a class or as a circuit/interval workout alternating 3 minutes of step and 1–1½ minutes of strength training.

### Squat with tricep extension

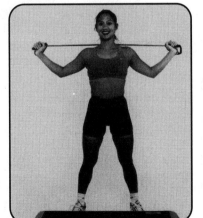
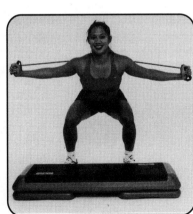

**Figure 8.28**

**Position:** Hold the tube behind your head.

**Action:** As you bend your knees, extend your arms to the side. As you stand up, bring arms back in to starting position.

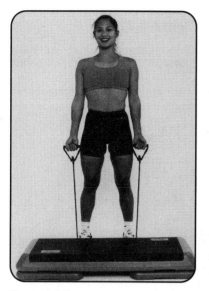

### Bicep curl with squat

**Position:** Position legs slightly wider than shoulder-width apart with tube under both feet.

**Action:** As you bend at the knees and sit back, bend the arms at the elbows.

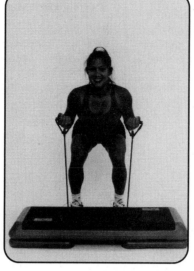

**Figure 8.29**

### Side lunge
### with single arm cross-over

**Position:** Stand with the tube under one foot on the step.

**Action:** Keep a slight bend at the elbow, and bring your outside arm across the midline of the body toward the opposite hip.

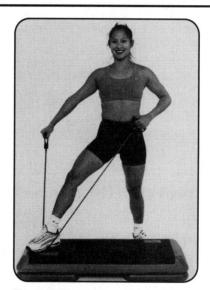

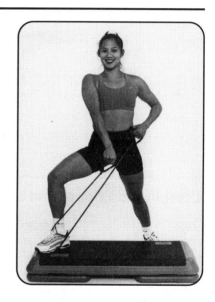

**Figure 8.30**

### Row with squat

**Position:** Place legs slightly wider than shoulder-width apart with the tube under both feet. Cross the tube handles.

**Action:** As you bend at the knees and sit back, pull elbows up and back and lift hands to chest level.

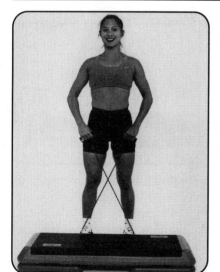

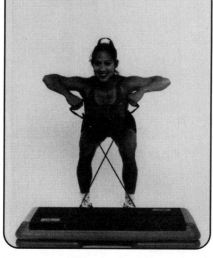

**Figure 8.31**

## Shoulder press with lunge

**Position:** Place the tube under your back foot and other foot on the step. Hold tube in hands at shoulder level.

**Action:** As you lunge down, lift arms over head.

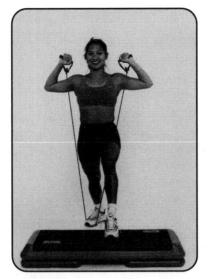
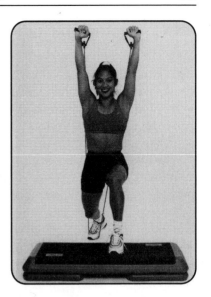

**Figure 8.32**

## Squat with leg abduction

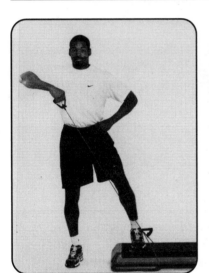
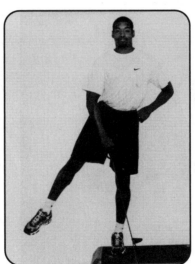

**Figure 8.33**

**Position:** Place the tube under the step and put one handle through the other handle. Stand to the side of the step with one foot on the step. As you squat, lift your arm to the side.

**Action:** As you lower your arm, shift your weight to the leg on the step and lift and abduct the other leg.

## Hamstring curl and front raise

**Position:** Make a loop with the tube by placing one handle through the other. Put one foot through the loop and place it around your ankle. Hold the other end of the tube in the opposite hand and stand on the tube (when lifting your left arm, step on tube with left foot and loop around right ankle).

**Action:** As you lift your arm to the front, bring your heel to your seat by bending your knee.

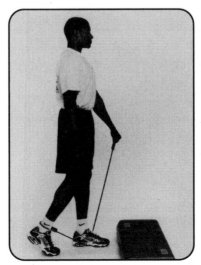
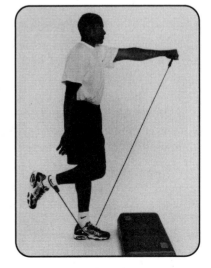

**Figure 8.34**

## ◼ **Step and Strength Intervals**

Step and strength intervals combine step aerobics with strength training using light resistance (tubing, resistance bands, or hand-held weights), performed in a unique interval-training format. This option produces an excellent total fitness workout in a short time.

The interval training workout follows this format: 3 minutes of high-intensity step aerobics conditioning (Figure 8.35), followed immediately by 1 minute of strength training using the bench and resistance equipment described earlier (Figure 8.36).

These 3-minute/1-minute intervals are repeated at least five times in a complete high-intensity workout time of 20 minutes, during which your heart rate is kept in the training zone.

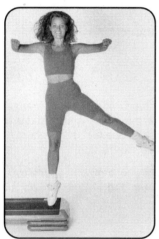 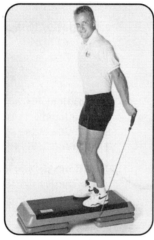

**Figure 8.35** Step and strength intervals — high-intensity step aerobics conditioning (3 minutes).

**Figure 8.36** Step and strength intervals — bench and resistance equipment (1 minute).

For safety, place the tubing (or resistance bands/hand-weights) under the bench. After your warm-up (see Chapter 4), do the first interval of step aerobics for 3 minutes. Then pick up the tubing and secure its position under the bench block's ends or under the center of the platform, whichever the exercise requires.

Perform the strength move by first positioning your feet comfortably apart, either a bit astride or side-by-side. Then with an exhale, press, and hold while you maximally contract the muscles used. Every time you perform against resistance, use your mind as well as your body to achieve the full contraction. Telling yourself "up-sque-e-e-ze-and-*hold*" helps to attain the full contraction. Return to the original position with an inhale ("and-relax"), breathing every time and continually.

While you press against resistance, maintain a little "squat," or *bending of the knees*, to keep the heart rate elevated and stay aerobic (continually using oxygen for your energy needs). To make sure you challenge yourself to perform to your maximum during every interval, take several "active recovery" heart rate checks during the 20 minutes. This will ensure that you are staying within your target heart rate zone at all times.

If you become fatigued during the strength interval, take a break or bring your arms up into position just halfway. Because step aerobics is lower-body intensive and these muscles get a big workout, *the strength interval focuses only on the muscles of the upper body.*

After the strength interval, replace the tubing (bands, weights) safely under the bench and perform the next step aerobics interval, continuing with this interval format for a minimum of 20 minutes.

> *Step and strength is an extremely popular method of accomplishing a complete workout in one location in minimum time, using an easily planned program routine. It is especially helpful during times in your life when you don't have much time to fitness-train.*

## SUMMARY

Strength training is another way of adding variation to your step aerobics program. This chapter presented more than a dozen exercises primarily targeting isolated muscle groups in the upper and middle body. All of these can involve using a variety of resistance equipment with the step/bench. The exercise prescription for strength training established by the ACSM is the basis for the underlying principles and guidelines.

Begin strength training slowly, methodically, and in absolute control of the amount of resistance or weights you are using. You will progress by increasing the resistance over time. You should record the exercises you perform, plus the number of sets, repetitions, and the type and amount of resistance used with each exercise. (Many of the exercises are shown with tubing, but the exercises also can be done using resistance bands or hand-weights.) Charting your progress in your Fitness Journal will give you a visual blueprint for success and a means of continual motivation.

Strength-fitness training to more fully develop muscle strength and endurance is a long-term project[14] calling for a dedicated personal commitment of many hours, just as the programs of stretching for flexibility improvement and step training for aerobic capacity improvement are. All fitness programs are for life.

# SECTION 2

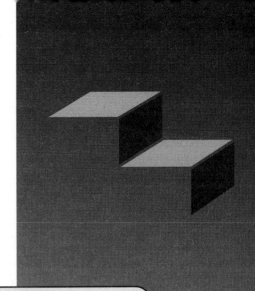

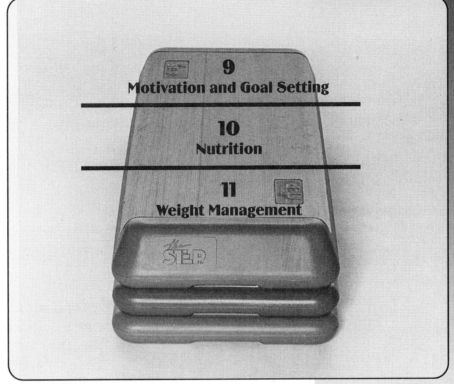

**9**
Motivation and Goal Setting

**10**
Nutrition

**11**
Weight Management

## ▰ The "Plus"

Section II addresses additional areas of awareness that one needs to consider when developing and following through with a total fitness program. It contains the "balancing steps" for healthy choices. The chapters in this section are listed above.

As you embark on Section 2, Chapters 9–11, you'll discover that you are in one of two categories of thinking, or "fitness mindsets":

1. An *acknowledged novice* to this idea of lifetime total fitness and (as the Introduction states) you realize that you need to be convinced that you are

going to *enjoy* beginning, and will *enjoy* continuing, a physically active lifestyle on a regular basis. You're choosing to begin the course here, in Chapter 9.

or

2. You have *already begun* the course, taking the necessary *steps in the right direction* by educating yourself to the concept of total fitness, have experienced the *first step* (which was understanding your starting points), have realized the *next step* was to become an informed and safe stepper, and have clarified what the *segments* of a step class are. You have traveled *step-by-step* and have learned many techniques, have creatively designed

how and where to *step rhythmically to the beat,* and have taken the *steps ahead,* adding various options, class formats, and strength training to the step training basics. Your fitness journey is well under way at this time!

Whether you are in the former (encouragement needed to begin) or latter (ideas needed to continue for a lifetime) category, let's look at how you can be personally in charge of your own fitness mindset. Taking ownership of and responsibility for all of your choices is fun — and the natural next step to take.

Prepare now to take those *balancing steps,* incorporating steps for developing mental strategies to stay *motivated* and *set goals,* steps for ensuring a healthy balance between energy output/input through *positive eating strategies,* and steps for understanding your own body composition followed by goal setting to achieve or maintain a healthy weight through *positive weight management* techniques.

Remember to continually journal and evaluate your progress. This provides a continual reminder that you *can* accomplish total fitness and enjoy the process, one successful step at a time!

As you begin Section II, ask yourself these questions.
Then check a response you're saying to yourself.

**9 Motivation and Goal Setting:**
Am I motivated to begin and continue
a total fitness program for life?
Motivated ☐
Need help with this one ☐

**10 Nutrition:**
Do I "eat and drink the
pyramids" in
nutrient-dense ways?
Yes ☐
No — what's that? ☐

**11 Weight Management:**
I understand body composition,
my own healthy weight, and
have a positive self-image.
Yes ☐ No ☐

*To the possession of the self,
the way is inward. (Plotinus)
We each must, therefore,
come of age by ourself.
Each must journey to find
our true center, alone.*

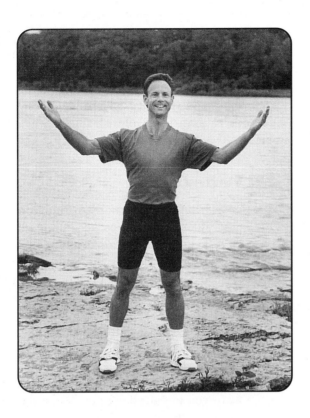

Finding the courage to change
is no more difficult than
learning to make one small
choice at a time.

*Choices,* Shad Helmstetter

To develop a mindset for enjoying living a fitness lifestyle, you first must become aware of how you make the choices you're currently making and, more specifically, *what internal resources you're using to make these choices.* Even though you can directly experience the results of your choices, you probably are unaware of the internal process used that led you to make your choices.

Awareness of this internal process is key to making new, more positive choices, for making all subsequent changes last a lifetime, and more important, *enjoying* the journey! The end result is that your mindset, or thinking, changes.

## ▨ Taking A Risk

Taking risks and embarking on something new requires courage. Changing physical fitness status is a case in point. To be open to identifying your medical history to yourself and others is difficult. To take the risk of receiving pretesting results you don't really want to know (because you have a feeling they are not what you're going to want to hear) is hard. To be open to suggestions on how to significantly change an unhealthy lifestyle that has become quite comfortable takes a significant act of courage.

You have enrolled in this fitness course, so celebrate the decision you have already made — that first, small choice. You're on your way! The first step is behind you. If you approach becoming fit with an "eating-the-elephant-one-bite-at-a-time" mindset, each choice (each "bite") will be digested easily and become a part of you. This proactive, planned approach combined with consistent practice will become a lifestyle change that lasts.

Individuals who have a quick-fix/lose-fat-in-a-few-weeks, reactionary mindset and a need for instant results usually become impatient with their progress. They will do too much too soon, incur injuries, or lower their resistance and physically "choke" on the big bite they're trying to take all at once.

Which is your mindset? If it is the latter, reframing it (thinking about it differently) as a methodical, proactive (planned) approach provides you with the opportunity to experience lasting results. Successes come continually when change is a one-small-choice-at-a-time process instead of one-big-end result. Celebrate your decision to change, and feel good about this one small choice. Then have patience with yourself, stay open-minded to ideas that are presented for you to consider, and enjoy the *process* of change that is now happening within you.

## Moving Out of Your Comfort Zone

Define to yourself: **What are the reasons that have moved me out of my comfort zone and motivated me to take that first step, that one small choice, toward fitness?** This is accomplished internally by forming *visual* pictures in your head, listening to what you're *saying* to yourself, or connecting with how you *feel* about your physical fitness status. Do you see/taste/smell/hear/feel (experience somehow) that you:

— can't keep up and are out-of-breath while trying to accomplish everyday physical tasks?

— choose to look better cosmetically and be more attractive to yourself and others?

— have a physical ailment that you know is present because you haven't taken care of yourself?

— now choose to be the best physical specimen of a human being you can possibly become?

— _____

— _____.

Immediately write down the reasons you pictured specifically or heard yourself say or felt within yourself. These sensory descriptions are the pleasure-seeking or pain-avoiding reasons that are motivating you! The goals you set will require you to choose methods to gain these pleasures or to avoid these pains.

## Motivation

True motivation lies internally within each of us. Once you identify the pleasure you're seeking or pain you're avoiding, you can request assistance externally, from other people or your environment, to temporarily coach and support your decision. Instructors, classmates, best friends, and attractive workout settings can give you the immediate information, encouragement, and gratification you need to get started or continue on your fitness journey for a lifetime.

No one can be with you for all 1,440 minutes available to you in your day to make the choices that reflect upon your fitness. Therefore, other people and your environment can be only temporary motivators in your lifetime fitness journey, because they are all external to you. It's the "kleenex analogy."[1] Use them when you need to. Then discard them and carry on!

*True motivation and lasting change have to be developed or happen internally.* This type of motivation is not difficult to acquire. Your internal coach is there just waiting to be called upon.[2] Internal motivation is simply a matter of understanding *how* to use your vast internal resources.

> *Your internal resources are thoughts reflecting*
> *— past and present life experiences*
> *— past present, and future needs, wants, and goals.[3]*

### What Are My Internal Resources?

You can use your internal resources to empower you when you need motivation, or to give you ideas on how to or how not to set your physical fitness goals.

Defining what these resources are within you will give you the key to accessing and enhancing your future and provide you with the ability to set powerful goals. These resources consist of your:

- Hereditary and environmental influences
- Positive and negative life experiences
- Wants, needs, priorities. and goals
- Strengths, talents, and interests
- Weaknesses, risk factors and poor choices
- Beliefs/truths/rules you follow
- Attitudes (interpreting an experience as positive or negative
- Feelings (emotions)
- Actions/behaviors/choices you have expressed (resulting from all of the above)

Take a contemplative moment and review these points. What mental pictures, self-talk, and feelings surface as thoughts reflecting your life experiences, needs, wants and goals? In terms of your physical fitness, the resources that surface will represent pleasureful or painful memories — thoughts with resulting actions that you'll choose to experience again and ones you don't choose to experience ever again!

*Moving toward pleasure-based results and away from painful ones are the forces behind motivation.* The direction you've just stated (toward pleasure or away from pain) reflects *how* you've stored your internal resources.

## How Internal Resources Affect Motivation

*How* have you stored your thoughts (internal resources) sensory-wise regarding your physical fitness? Do you remember an earlier attempt at step training, aerobics, fitness walking, strength training, or stretching as a positive experience that met your goal at the time? How do you picture, hear, taste, smell, self-talk, and feel about that experience? You might say, "Great workout! I was energized and made lots of friends!" or "The room smelled terrible; I'll never go back there!"

What answers your thoughts are your *sensory representations*. Visual pictures, sounds, feelings, or smells come to mind. You can hear yourself stating the two examples just given. A feeling comes over you that is either pleasant or painful. Motivation, thus, has the following sensory components:

- Images, sounds, tastes, smell
- Internal self-talk
- Body sensations (movements, touch, emotions).

## IMAGES, SOUNDS, TASTES, SMELLS

Individuals should take ownership of, or responsibility for, how they are picturing or imaging the fitness goals they're choosing to set. Images that are big, bright, in color, and moving are more powerful than small, dim, black-and-white, freeze-frame images. The same applies to tastes, sounds, and smells. They are fresh or tangy, soft or loud, strong or weak. Ask yourself: "How *large* are the images I'm making in my head? Are they small like a postcard or large as a poster?" (Figure 9.1). More powerful images are more motivating. Goals established with powerful images will be accomplished much more quickly.

## SELF-TALK

Internal dialogue that is in the present tense, positive, and enabling is more motivating than self-talk that is in the past tense or future tense, negative, and disabling, For example, "I am confident of my ability to learn new step training moves quickly and am enjoying my instructor's creative, improvising style" is more powerful and motivating than stating to one's self, "I will feel confident of my ability in step training class as soon as I learn all the basic moves and get to know the instructor." Listen to the verbs and adverbs in your sentences, and construct talk that is *as if it's already accomplished.*

## BODY SENSATIONS

Body sensations that focus on gaining pleasure instead of avoiding pain ("doing my best" instead of "not tripping over the bench") and sensations that are quick, powerful, big high, and the like are important to make because they tell your brain *how to*

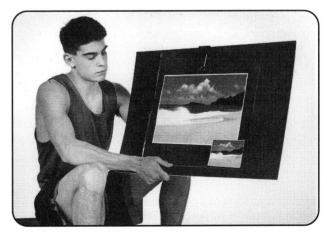

**Figure 9.1** How large are the images I'm making in my head? Are they small like a postcard or large as a poster?"

do something. For example, if you want to get up in the morning and are lying in the comfort of bed, what will motivate you to get up? Actually, what *did* motivate you to get up at 6:30 a.m. on a Saturday morning this past winter? Did you:

— picture how cold, gray, and dreary it was outside,

— say, "Gosh, it's so *early*, and I'm so *tired*," and

— slowly move out of bed?

or did you:

— picture, taste, smell a fun event you had planned for the day,

— say to yourself, "It's great to be alive! Today is a fresh new day with no mistakes!" and

— spring up quickly?

> *If you're not motivated to do something you must change your images, tastes, sounds, smells, self-talk, movements, touch and feelings. It's that simple.*

### KEEPING THE POWER TO CHANGE

To use your full potential to set powerful goals, you must take ownership of your internal resources. This requires you to take responsibility and not blame others or the environment for your successes and failures. Retaining ownership of your total fitness program goals provides you with the ability to change, to set powerful goals that *you* choose, and to go about the business of systematically achieving them.

If a goal you're setting for yourself doesn't happen soon enough, and any type of blame enters the internal picturing, feelings, and self-talk, stop. Take ownership and state: "I own this situation. How can I get the results I need? How can I repicture or talk differently about this situation so it is helpful to me?" Taking ownership of your internal resources — your thoughts — is the key to personal freedom and to all goal achievement. You have a free will and are in charge of your life. Enjoy the freedom and choose wisely, one small choice at a time!

## ■ Goal-Setting Strategies

It's time to apply your new knowledge of internal motivation and plan your future by first acknowledging,

and perhaps reestablishing, your time priorities, so you can set powerful goals.

### Establishing Priorities

Priorities refer to how you spend your time, and are the "means" to reach your goals (the "ends" you seek). You can use Exercise 9.1 to set your top 20 priorities. It allows you to identify how many hours per day and week you devote to each priority, and to record time robbers that take you away from a priority.

Can you identify an excellent role model whom you associate with each? Positive role models provide us time-saving, short-cut ideas on how to do something the quickest, most efficient, and best way possible. Take advantage of their strategies whenever possible by taking a risk and asking them *how* they do what they do.

In the last column of the figure, you can rank each priority by how you now feel about it (not which takes the most time). The key to setting powerful fitness goals is to be certain that *your time has been prioritized or is being prioritized* to include these goals you've set, to enable them to happen.

### Creating the Future in Advance

The foundation for successful goal setting has just been established, as follows:

1. Identifying *reasons* you're choosing to change

2. Becoming aware of how you're motivated — which senses are used and how — and, consequently, how to change your actions at the sensory-thought level

3. Assessing and reestablishing your time priorities, to enable change to happen.

Now it's time to set some goals. This goal-setting procedure tells your brain precisely what goal you are choosing to set. It provides solid (positive, pleasure) reasoning for why you're choosing this goal. It then breaks old programming by stating all of your negative pain-avoidance reasons. Heap them on big here. Make it *painful* to continue to make poor choices. Immediate positive-action choices are then made to create the motivational pictures, self-talk, and movements necessary to initiate active change in your program, starting this moment.

Do you need more help? Try making an audiotape! Making an audiotape of yourself responding to the statements and questions for each goal you set may prove extremely helpful. You'll find that the repetition of this blueprinting process is a unique time short-cut to achieving your goals. During the goal-setting process, one end to keep in mind is to have *fun* during your pursuit of fitness!

## SUMMARY

A sample goal-setting page, Exercise 9.2, is provided here for you to develop your skills. Begin the practice of constructing goals by writing one of your own right now. Setting goals helps to keep you

focused daily on improvement and positive change. It encourages consistency in your fitness program and helps to keep you on target. Without goals, there's nothing to shoot for!

When they are properly set internally and nourished continually, goals become reality. Believe it, and you will see it. Your future resides within you as a rich resource of possibilities.

> One simple decision:
>   consciously
>     actively
>       make your choices.
>             *Choices*, Shad Helmstetter

## Exercise 9.1  Establishing Time Priorities

Priorities are the means to your ends. They are things you give time to in the wellness dimension areas of your life: physical/social/emotional/spiritual/intellectual/talent expression.

| Top 20 Priorities (Listed in any order) | Hours Each Day | Hours Each Week | Time Robbers | Role Model | Rank Order of Importance |
|---|---|---|---|---|---|
| ▮ | | | | | # |
| ▮ | | | | | # |
| ▮ | | | | | # |
| ▮ | | | | | # |
| ▮ | | | | | # |
| ▮ | | | | | # |
| ▮ | | | | | # |
| ▮ | | | | | # |
| ▮ | | | | | # |
| ▮ | | | | | # |
| ▮ | | | | | # |
| ▮ | | | | | # |
| ▮ | | | | | # |
| ▮ | | | | | # |
| ▮ | | | | | # |
| ▮ | | | | | # |
| ▮ | | | | | # |
| ▮ | | | | | # |
| ▮ | | | | | # |
| ▮ | | | | | # |

## Exercise 9.2 Developing Goal Scripts

For every goal you'll ever set, consider the following four statements and questions. *Using one or several full sentences* for each step, write down your immediate responses in the spaces provided. All of the responses to these four segments of a goal, collectively, become one goal or "goal script" — the precise language you'll repeat to yourself at least twice daily until you achieve the goal.

**Write One Complete Goal ("Goal Script")**

❶ **State one goal in positive, *present-tense* language. Ask yourself, "What will I experience — see, hear, taste, smell, feel — when I achieve it?" You'll recognize these as the components of motivation. All powerful goals use the SMART formula: specific, measurable, achievable, realistic, timely.** *Example:* "I am choosing to become physically fit within the next 10 weeks by practicing everything I learn in class for 2–4 additional times every week. This goal encourages me because I am able to continually breathe easier in all activities I do. I feel a new sense of discipline and in charge of my life, and I project a healthier image because I am continually dropping 1–2 unnecessary fat pounds per week."

STEP 1

❷ **State your *pleasure-value reasons*. Ask yourself, "Why am I totally committed to achieving each goal?" Involve your positive, "moving toward" values to answer this question. Values may be any of the following: adventure and change, commitment, freedom, giving pleasure to others, happiness, health, love, power, prestige and worth, security, life purpose, success, expression of talent, trust, loyalty, and any other positive values important to you.** *Example:* "Having this goal and continually working on it proves I am able to make and keep *commitments* to myself."

STEP 2

❸ **State your *pain-avoidance value reasons*. Because we do more to avoid pain than to gain pleasure, heap on the painful thoughts so you're really motivated to change! Break the link of the old programmed ways by asking yourself, "What painful values do I choose to avoid?" Some pain-avoidance values are: anger, resentment, anxiety, worry, boredom, depression, embarrassment, frustration, guilt, humiliation, jealousy, feeling overwhelmed, physical pain, prejudice, rejection, sadness.** *Example:* "If I don't continually work on this goal I've set I'll feel *angry, guilty,* and *depressed* at myself that I can't follow through on something that is extremely important to me at this time of my life. Why would I choose to continually feel this way?!"

STEP 3

❹ **Reestablish the pleasure link by picturing, hearing feeling, "What *actions* do I choose to take or do immediately to master this goal? What is something I can start doing right now and within the next 24 hours?"** *Example:* "I choose to practice all of the physical fitness moves presented in class this term at least every other day, and for 40 continuous minutes per session. In addition, I choose to continually be aware of all the mental training aspects I am learning and incorporate them into my daily total fitness program."

STEP 4

This is your entire goal, stated in the form of a script of motivational language, that you alone have personally chosen. This is the format used by individuals both in the professional world and private sector who daily achieve excellence, success, — and their goals!

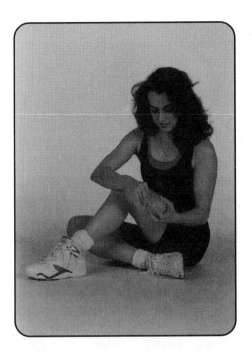

Choose what is best;
habit will soon render it
agreeable and easy

    — Pythagoras

This ancient principle for making choices hasn't really changed today. Better or best choices are always available for you to make. The actions you take reflect whether you simply have the knowledge or whether you *apply* the knowledge. Enjoy making the best available choices, all day long.

## ■ Nutrients for Going and Growing

Your body needs two basic types of nutrients:

1. Foods that satisfy your energy needs.
2. Foods that meet your needs for growth, repair, and regulation of body processes.

*Nutrients* are chemical substances that your body absorbs from food during digestion. Your body needs at least 40 nutrients.

*Essential nutrients* are those your body cannot make or is unable to make in adequate amounts. These nutrients must be obtained from what you eat and drink. If your diet does not provide them properly, your body cannot perform well, mentally or physically.

This is where choice comes in. You may know what the better choices of foods are (called *nutrient-dense* foods[1]), but if you don't eat the best choices available to you, you really don't practice good nutrition at all. Good health, optimum fitness, and good nutrition result from not just knowing what is best but actually choosing it 80% to 90% of the time.[2]

*Diet* here means *total intake of food and drink*. A well-balanced diet is one that contains these six basic nutrients:

1. Carbohydrates      4. Vitamins
2. Fats               5. Minerals
3. Proteins           6. Water

## ◼ Dietary Plans

Proper amounts of each are established according to your age, gender, activity level, and state of wellness. These nutrients can be supplied from eating and fluid replacement plans such as those presented here:

◼ *Food Guide Pyramid.* A Guide to Daily Food Choices, established by the U. S. Department of Agriculture[3] and shown in Figure 10.1, depicting the major food groups;

◼ *Pyramid Plus.* A Star-Studded Guide to Food Choices for Better Health,[4] published by the Oregon Dairy Council, listing nutrient density information throughout the chapter and shown in Figure 10.3 depicting the number and size of servings recommended.

◼ *Food Guide Pyramid for Vegetarian Meal Planning*[5], (Figure 10.4).

◼ *Fluid Replacement Pyramid*[6, 7] (Figure 10.5).

You cannot always take in all of the essential nutrients every 24 hours. What *is* important is that over a span of several days and weeks, you continually select from the five groups to meet your nutrient needs. The pyramids *outline* what to eat each day. They are not rigid prescriptions but, rather, general guides that let you choose a healthful diet that's right for you. The pyramids call for eating a variety of foods to get the nutrients you need and, at the same time, the proper amount of calories to maintain a healthy weight.

The Food Guide Pyramid focuses on fat because most U. S. diets are too high in fat, especially saturated fat. The pyramid emphasizes foods from the five major food groups shown in the three lower sections of the pyramid. Each of these food groups provides some, but not all, of the nutrients you need. Foods in one group can't replace those in another. No one food group is more important than another. For good health, you need them all.

## Nutrient Density

Following the description of each food group, next, foods are listed according to *nutrient density, the amount of nutrition per calorie each food provides.*[8] Choose foods from the four-star groups (Figure 10.2) since they provide the most nutrition for the least calories. The categories are:[9]

4 stars = most nutrition per calorie

3 stars = next to most nutrition per calorie

2 stars = next to least nutrition per calorie

1 star = least nutrition per calorie.

They are also ranked *within* each starred group, and listed in descending order of nutrients per calorie.[9]

### MILK AND MILK PRODUCTS GROUP

*Calcium,* riboflavin (vitamin B$_2$), and protein are the key nutrients needed to build the basic structure and strength of bones and teeth, assist in the production of energy needs, and help in the growth and maintenance of every living cell. If you are not an avid milk fan, other foods in the milk and milk products group (Table 10.1), will supply the calcium, riboflavin, and protein you need.

### TABLE 10.1    Ratings of Milk and Milk Products

| Rating: | Food Choices in Ranked Order for Calcium |
|---|---|
| ★ | nonfat plain yogurt |
| ★ | nonfat milk |
| ★ | nonfat cream cheese |
| ★ | 1% milk |
| | buttermilk |
| | lowfat cheese |
| | 2% milk |
| ★ | part-skim ricotta cheese |
| ★ | whole milk |
| ★ | regular fat cheese |
| | lowfat chocolate milk |
| | lowfat fruit yogurt |
| | nonfat frozen yogurt |
| ★ | pudding |
| ★ | custard |
| | lowfat frozen yogurt |
| | ice milk |
| ★ | milkshake |
| | cottage cheese |
| | ice cream |
| | nonfat sour cream |

# Food Guide Pyramid
## A Guide to Daily Food Choices

**KEY**

● Fat (naturally occurring and added)

▶ Sugars (added)

These symbols show fat and added sugars in foods.

The small tip of the pyramid shows fats, oils, and sweets. These are foods such as salad dressings and oils, cream, butter, margarine, sugars, soft drinks, candies, and sweet desserts. These foods provide calories and little else nutritionally. Most people should use them sparingly.

The next level of the Food Guide Pyramid has two groups of foods that come mostly from animals: milk, yogurt, and cheese; and meat, poultry, fish, dry beans, eggs, and nuts. These foods are important sources of protein, calcium, iron, and zinc.

The next level includes foods that come from plants — vegetables and fruits. Most people need to eat more of these foods for the vitamins, minerals, and fiber they supply.

At the base of the Food Guide Pyramid are breads, cereals, rice, and pasta — all foods from grains. You need the most servings of these foods each day.

Fats, Oils, & Sweets
**USE SPARINGLY**

Milk, Yogurt, & Cheese Group
**2-3 SERVINGS**

Meat, Poultry, Fish, Dry Beans, Eggs, & Nuts Group
**2-3 SERVINGS**

Vegetable Group
**3-5 SERVINGS**

Fruit Group
**2-4 SERVINGS**

Bread, Cereal, Rice, & Pasta Group
**6-11 SERVINGS**

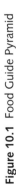

Source: U. S. Department of Agriculture

**Figure 10.1** Food Guide Pyramid

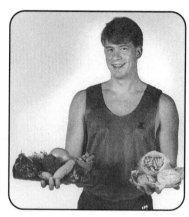

**Figure 10.2** Choose nutrient-dense foods over calorie-dense foods.

## MEAT AND MEAT ALTERNATIVES GROUP

Key nutrients in this group are *iron, protein,* niacin, thiamin, zinc, and vitamin $B_2$. Even though this group is sometimes called simply the "meat group," plant foods, when eaten together, can supply the needed protein, niacin, iron, and thiamine and are considered an alternative to eating meat (Table 10.2). (In fact, a separate eating plan for these person's choosing to eat only "alternatives to meat" is included following the Pyramid Plus starred eating plan.) Some

of the plant foods that can be combined, enabling their proteins to complement each other (allow the amino acids to combine to form balanced protein), are dried beans and whole wheat, dried beans and corn or rice, and peanuts and wheat.[10]

One serving is equal to 2–3 ounces of cooked lean meat, fish, or poultry, or the protein equivalent. Visually, a 2- to 3-ounce portion fills the palm of an average hand and is the width of the little finger. All excess fat should be removed from any meat you eat. You should remove the skin from poultry and eat only the meat, eliminating unnecessary calories.

## VEGETABLE GROUP

Key nutrients are *folic acid, vitamins A and C,* which are catalysts or action starters, and fiber (Table 10.3). Their most important functions are:

- Form and maintain skin and body linings
- Cement substances to promote strength in cells and hasten healing of injuries
- Function in all visual processes
- Aid in the use of iron.

**Sources of Vitamin A**     Remembering two simple colors — orange and green — will remind you that

**TABLE 10.2     Ratings of Meat and Meat Alternatives**

| Rating: | Food Choices in Ranked Order for Iron and Protein |
|---|---|
| ★ | fish, shellfish |
| ★ | poultry (light meat, skinless) |
| ★ | turkey ham |
| ★ | beef (round and sirloin, well-trimmed) |
| | pork (tenderloin, well-trimmed) |
| | veal (leg and shoulder, well-trimmed) |
| | lentils |
| ★ | beef (rib, chuck, flank and ground) |
| ★ | ham (lean) |
| ★ | tofu |
| | veal and lamb (leg and loin) |
| | poultry (dark meat with skin) |
| | pork (loin and rib) |
| | Canadian bacon |
| | poultry sausage |
| | dried beans and peas |
| | eggs |
| ★ | hot dogs |
| ★ | pork sausage |
| | chicken nuggets |
| | fish sticks |
| | nuts and seeds |
| ★ | peanut butter |
| | bologna |

**TABLE 10.3     Ratings for Vegetable Group**

| Rating: | Food Choices in Ranked Order for Folic Acid and Vitamins A and C* |
|---|---|
| ★ | red and green bell peppers |
| ★ | bok choy |
| ★ | spinach |
| ★ | leaf lettuce |
| | broccoli |
| | carrots |
| | cauliflower |
| ★ | cabbage, chard |
| ★ | asparagus, kale |
| ★ | vegetable juice, brussels sprouts |
| | iceberg lettuce, sweet potato |
| | tomato, snow peas |
| | zucchini, okra |
| | winter squash, green beans |
| ★ | beets, cucumber |
| ★ | celery, jicama |
| | artichoke, peas |
| | mushrooms |
| ★ | eggplant, corn |
| | avocado, potato |

*Based on 100-calorie portions.

foods of these colors provide vitamin A. You should eat dark green, leafy, and orange vegetables (such as carrots, sweet potatoes, and greens) regularly. Because vitamin A is stored in the fat tissue of the body, an overdose through supplementation in pill form can be fatal. (The same is true for the other fat-soluble vitamins — D, E, and K.)

**Sources of Vitamin C**  Daily servings of vegetables such as broccoli, bell peppers, and spinach are recommended for supplying the needed catalyst vitamin C. This vitamin is water-soluble, which means that if you take in too much, the excess is excreted through the urine. If you decide to take vitamin C supplement pills in massive doses, your body will react by increasing the level it needs. If you then stop taking vitamin C supplements suddenly, your body will react as if it were deficient! Supplementation is costly and unnecessary for well people who eat properly.

## FRUIT GROUP

Key ingredients are *folic acid, vitamins A and C,* and fiber (Table 10.4).

## BREADS AND CEREALS GROUP

Your number-one daily need is energy to perform every daily function from sleeping to step aerobics. Although the breads and cereals group assists with the growth and maintenance of cells and with the elimination process (fiber provides bulk to your waste for easy removal), the major function is to provide *energy*.

If you do not use this carbohydrate food for the expenditure of energy, for growth and repair, or eliminate it, you wear it as body fat — future energy. It's like constantly carrying around extra gasoline for your car. If you are an active person, such as a varsity or endurance athlete, you will want to provide an abundance of this energy food.

Key ingredients are *fiber, complex carbohydrates,* thiamine, iron, and niacin (Table 10.5).

## "SOMETIMES" FOODS

The foods classified as extras or "sometimes" have no recommended number of servings. These foods

### TABLE 10.4  Ratings for Fruit Group

| Rating: | Food Choices in Ranked Order for Folic Acid and Vitamins A and C |
|---|---|
| ★ | papaya |
| ★ | strawberries |
| ★ | kiwi |
| ★ | orange, grapefruit |
| | orange juice |
| | cantaloupe |
| | mandarin oranges |
| | mango |
| ★ | honeydew (melon) |
| ★ | raspberries |
| ★ | apricots |
| | rhubarb |
| | pineapple |
| | watermelon |
| | pineapple juice |
| | blueberries |
| ★ | peach |
| ★ | banana |
| | plum |
| | cherries |
| | frozen fruit |
| | juice bar |
| | canned fruit |
| ★ | pears |
| | apples |
| | dried fruit |
| | grapes |
| | raisins |

### TABLE 10.5  Ratings for Breads and Cereals Group

| Rating: | Food Choices in Ranked Order for Fiber and Complex Carbohydrates |
|---|---|
| ★ | barley |
| ★ | bulgur |
| ★ | bran or whole-grain cereals |
| ★ | popcorn (air-popped or lite microwave) |
| | whole-grain breads |
| | oatmeal |
| | whole-grain pasta |
| | corn or whole-wheat tortilla |
| ★ | brown rice |
| ★ | bran muffin |
| ★ | whole-grain crackers |
| | soft pretzel or breadstick |
| | English muffin |
| | enriched pasta |
| | popcorn (oil-popped) |
| ★ | flour tortilla, bagel |
| ★ | enriched breads, enriched rice |
| | pancakes, waffles |
| | graham crackers, saltines |
| | sweetened cereal |
| | dry pretzels or breadsticks |
| ★ | cornbread |
| | fruit or nut bread |
| | biscuit, stuffing |
| | croissant |

provide little nutrition and often are high in sugar, salt, fat, and calories. Classified as extras are:

| | | |
|---|---|---|
| bacon | french fries | pickles |
| bouillon | fruit-flavored | pies |
| butter |   drinks | potato chips |
| cakes | gelatin dessert | salad dressings |
| candy | gravy | sauces |
| coffee | honey | seasonings |
| condiments | jam | sherbet |
| cookies | jelly | soft drinks |
| snack crackers | margarine | sour cream |
| cream | mayonnaise | sugar |
| regular fat cream | nondairy creamer | tea |
|   cheese | olives | tortilla chips |
| doughnuts | onion rings | vegetable oils[11] |

## SERVINGS PER DAY?[12]

The ranges given in Figure 10.3 are guides for how much food to eat each day. *Choose the lower or higher number of servings based on your caloric needs.* If you eat more or less than one serving, count as partial servings. For children under age 5, a serving is ¼–½ of a standard serving. To get enough calcium, however, all children need a total of at least two standard servings of milk or milk products each day.

The number of servings you need depends on how many calories you need, which in turn depends on your age, gender, physical condition, and how active you are. Almost everyone should have at least the

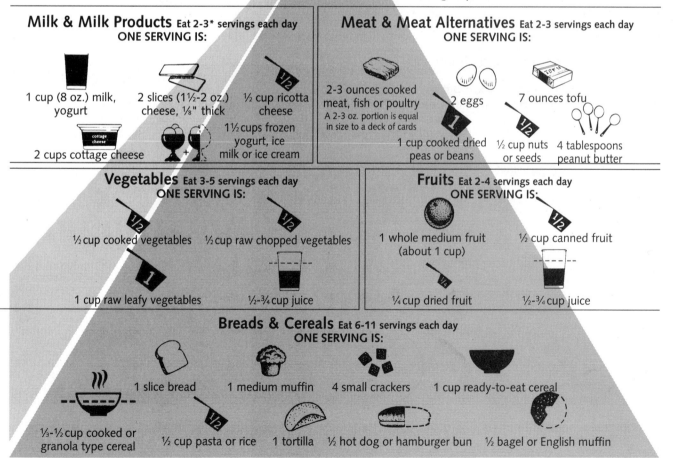

## How Many Servings Do You Need Each Day?

### Sometimes Foods
Sometimes foods provide little or no nutrition and are often high in fat, sugar, salt and calories. They should be eaten in moderation and not in place of servings from the five food groups.

**Milk & Milk Products** Eat 2-3* servings each day
ONE SERVING IS:

1 cup (8 oz.) milk, yogurt   2 slices (1½-2 oz.) cheese, ⅛" thick   ½ cup ricotta cheese
2 cups cottage cheese   1½ cups frozen yogurt, ice milk or ice cream

**Meat & Meat Alternatives** Eat 2-3 servings each day
ONE SERVING IS:

2-3 ounces cooked meat, fish or poultry
A 2-3 oz. portion is equal in size to a deck of cards
2 eggs   7 ounces tofu
1 cup cooked dried peas or beans   ½ cup nuts or seeds   4 tablespoons peanut butter

**Vegetables** Eat 3-5 servings each day
ONE SERVING IS:

½ cup cooked vegetables   ½ cup raw chopped vegetables
1 cup raw leafy vegetables   ½-¾ cup juice

**Fruits** Eat 2-4 servings each day
ONE SERVING IS:

1 whole medium fruit (about 1 cup)   ½ cup canned fruit
¼ cup dried fruit   ½-¾ cup juice

**Breads & Cereals** Eat 6-11 servings each day
ONE SERVING IS:

1 slice bread   1 medium muffin   4 small crackers   1 cup ready-to-eat cereal
⅓-½ cup cooked or granola type cereal   ½ cup pasta or rice   1 tortilla   ½ hot dog or hamburger bun   ½ bagel or English muffin

•Young Adults (9–18 years) and Older Adults (51+) need 4 servings

Source: Nutrition Education Services/Oregon Dairy Council, "Pyramid Plus" pamphlet (Portland, OR: Oregon Dairy Council, 1997).©

**Figure 10.3**

minimum number of servings from each of the five major food groups daily. Many women, older children, and most teenagers and men need more. The top of the range is about right for an active man or a teenage boy.

To apply the guidelines on servings to your specific needs, Table 10.6 provides "Sample Diets for a Day at Three Calorie Levels."[13,14]

## Alternative/Vegetarian Diets

Viable options are available and good choices can be made in every dimension of the lifetime fitness program you're designing for yourself. Your eating plan is no exception. The educational/research association of professional affiliates responsible for certifying registered dietitians and licensed nutritionists has published its latest position on an alternative eating plan you might also choose to consider, entitled, "Vegetarian Diets".[15]

To understand this acceptable alternative to eating the traditional food pyramid mentioned previously, it is suggested that you take the time now to assess yourself regarding the following three points. The detailed questions to ask yourself pertaining to each point is provided at the end of this chapter on Exercise 10.1 entitled, "Considerations for Vegetarian meal Planning":

1. Identify the *group(s)* you're choosing to eat in an alternative way (meat group, milk group, meat and milk groups, fats/oils/sweets group) and the *reason* for each choice.

2. Do you understand *what the required nutrients are* (that are provided in each group) that have to be considered and *replaced* by other forms of alternative food choices (that likewise can provide those required nutrients)?

3. Does this new choice of eating plan fulfill *your needs* regarding the six total wellness dimensions of your life?

Once you've assessed all of the needs you have regarding the complex topic of food and feeding yourself, it then is possible to proceed with considering an alternative eating plan.

Some research findings to consider are as follows:

- Studies are showing that a high animal-based diet is more likely to lead to heart disease, cancer, high blood pressure, diabetes, strokes, and obesity.[16]

- A plant-based diet is higher in vitamins and fiber, lower in cholesterol and other animal fats that may reduce or even reverse the risk of the aforementioned health risks.[17, 18]

- A *well-planned* vegetarian eating lifestyle can generally meet all of the nutrients required for energy, growth, and repair of tissues.[19, 20]

- If strict vegan diets (described in Exercise 10.1) are adopted or if you are in a special-needs group

## TABLE 10.6    Sample Diets for a Day at Three Calorie Levels.

|  | **About 1600** | **About 2200** | **About 2800** |
|---|---|---|---|
|  | 1600 calories is about right for many sedentary women and some older adults. | 2200 calories is about right for most children, teenage girls, active women, and many sedentary men. Women who are pregnant or breastfeeding may need somewhat more. | 2800 calories is about right for teenage boys, many active men, and some very active women. |
| Bread group servings | 6 | 9 | 11 |
| Fruit group servings | 2 | 3 | 4 |
| Vegetable group servings | 3 | 4 | 5 |
| Meat group | 5 ounces | 6 ounces | 7 ounces |
| Milk group servings | 2–3* | 2–3* | 2–3* |
| Total fat (grams)** | 53 | 73 | 93 |
| Total added sugars (teaspoons)** | 6 | 12 | 18 |

\* Women who are pregnant or breastfeeding, teenagers, and young adults to age 24 need 3 servings.

\*\* See bulletin on fat and cholesterol for more information on how to count fat. See bulletin on sugar for more information on sugars.

Source: U. S. Department of Agriculture, Human Nutrition Information Service, *Home and Garden Bulletin*, Number 253-2, p. 5, July 1993.

## Food Guide Pyramid for Vegetarian Meal Planning

**FATS, OILS, AND SWEETS — use sparingly**
Candy, butter, margarine, salad dressing, cooking oil

**MILK, YOGURT, AND CHEESE GROUP**
**0–3 servings daily***
milk — 1 cup
yogurt — 1 cup
natural cheese — 1½ oz.

*Vegetarians who choose not to use milk, yogurt, or cheese need to select other food sources rich in calcium. For a list of calcium-rich foods, please see Figure 1 on the 1997 American Dietetics Association Position Paper on Vegetarian Diets[22]

**DRY BEANS, NUTS, SEEDS, EGGS, AND MEAT SUBSTITUTES GROUP**
**2–3 servings daily**
soy milk — 1 cup
cooked dry beans or peas — ½ cup
1 egg or 2 egg whites
nuts or seeds — ⅓ cup
tofu or tempeh — ½ cup
peanut butter — 2 Tbsp

**VEGETABLE GROUP**
**3–5 servings daily**
cooked or chopped, raw
vegetables — ½ cup
raw, leafy vegetables — 1 cup

**FRUIT GROUP**
**2–4 servings daily**
juice — ¾ cup
dried fruit — ¼ cup
chopped, raw fruit — ½ cup
canned fruit — 1/2 cup
1 medium-size piece of fruit,
such as banana, apple, or orange

**BREAD, CEREAL, RICE, AND PASTA GROUP**
**6–11 servings daily**
bread — 1 slice
ready-to-eat cereal — 1 oz.
cooked cereal — ½ cup
cooked rice, pasta, or other grains — ½ cup
bagel — ½

Author(s): Title. Copyright The American Dietetic Association. Reprinted with permission from the *Journal of the American Dietetic Association*, Vol. 97; 1317–1321.

**Figure 10.4**   Food Guide Pyramid for Vegetarian Meal Planning

(pregnant, lactating, infant, child, or adolescent), you *must* consult with a registered dietitian or a licensed nutritionist. This certified professional is qualified to answer your alternative food-choice questions and is able to design an alternative eating plan program for your own special needs.

A variety of menu-planning approaches can provide vegetarians with adequate nutrition. The text version of the Food Guide Pyramid for Vegetarian Meal Planning is one approach.[21] In addition, the following guidelines can help vegetarians plan healthful diets.

■ Choose a variety of foods, including whole grains, vegetables, fruits, legumes, nuts, seeds and, if desired, dairy products and eggs.

■ Choose whole, unrefined foods often, and minimize intake of highly sweetened, fatty, and heavily refined foods.

■ Choose a variety of fruits and vegetables.

■ If animal foods such as dairy products and eggs are used, choose lower-fat versions of these foods. Cheeses and other high-fat dairy foods and eggs should be limited in the diet because of their saturated fat content and because their frequent use displaces plant foods in some vegetarian diets.

■ Vegans should include a regular source of vitamin $B_{12}$ in their diet along with a source of vitamin D if sun exposure is limited.

### Fluid Replacement Pyramid

Water is the best fluid for hydrating the body, especially when exercising for the duration of *up to* 60 to 90 continuous minutes.[23] In general, adults need 1 milliliter of water for every calorie expended. This formula converts into *6–8 cups per day*. To keep your body cool, more is required in warm weather and during exercise (see fluid replacement pyramid).

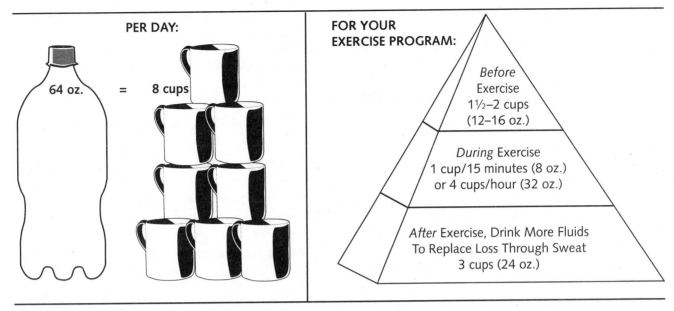

**Figure 10.5** Fluid Replacement Pyramid.

Some fluid replacement pointers are:[24, 25]

■ Adequate fluid intake hydrates the body and, in turn, enhances all performance and reduces the possibility of a heat stress illness.

■ Fluids should be consumed on a regular scheduled basis, not just when you get thirsty. Thirst usually reflects dehydration and a loss of important fluids and electrolytes.

■ When exercising for longer endurance periods (more than 90 continuous minutes), sports drinks may be considered a viable option to assist in replacement of important fluids and electrolytes.

■ The visual key to check if you are *adequately hydrating yourself*: clear, light-colored urine.

As an action plan for fluid replacement:

■ Measure out 64 oz. (8 cups) of water (Figure 10.5) and be sure to consume it all that day. This can be easily accomplished by continually refilling a sports squeeze bottle with this measured-out amount and taking it with you.

■ Drink water as your choice beverage for snacks, breaks, and meal-times.

■ Cooling alternatives: If you'd prefer a hydrating change to water, choose fluids with no caffeine or alcohol and little sugar or sodium. Consider any of these three alternatives:

— Mix 100% juice with plain or sparkling water.

— Mix unsweetened, decaffeinated iced tea with orange juice or lemonade.[26]

— Squeeze a wedge of lemon, lime, or orange into unflavored carbonated water, or add a mint sprig.

## Your Own Food Guide Pyramid

Considering *all* of the information presented in this chapter, develop in your Fitness Journal your own food guide pyramid for planning your meals, using a format similar to Figure 10.1. Design this *ideal* eating plan early in the course, to give yourself time to continually work at adjusting it to best fit all of your needs.

At the completion of the course, review your ideal food guide pyramid and, if necessary, redesign one then to include all of the new choices and changes you're incorporating into a permanent eating plan. It may help to post this final food guide pyramid eating plan on your refrigerator.

## Monitoring Food and Beverage Intake

Do you eat a wide variety of foods in moderation as shown in the U.S.D.A. Food Guide Pyramid described in detail in the "Pyramid Plus" starred food groups, or the ADA's Vegetarian Meal Planning guidelines?

After you have formulated your eating plan, think about what you have consumed today, and record the foods and beverages you ate and drank. Identify:

■ nutrient density starred ratings (4/3/2/1/0)

■ appropriate food group for each item

- size/quantity of serving
- with whom, where, why
- duration of time taken to eat
- other activity engaged in while eating
- Chapter 11 will request an additional entry, regarding your "felt senses", rating how full or empty you feel, before/during/after consumption.

A sample charting of these entries can be found on Figure 10.7, "Food and Beverage Intake Diary for One Day" provided at the end of this chapter. Record this information in your Fitness Journal.

For a combination food, think about what foods went into it and identify those foods with the appropriate food group. For example, the cheese on a pizza would be recorded in the Milk group, the tomatoes and any other vegetables in the Vegetable group, and the crust in the Breads group. The ingredients in a combination food may not always count as a full serving from the food group. Think in terms of quantity of servings, along with its nutrient category.

Continue monitoring your intake for at least one week. How does it measure up to the standards established for a balanced diet with special attention to selecting nutrient-dense foods? If your diet lacks variety, moderation, or foods from one of the food groups, you may not be getting all the nutrients and energy you need.

It's easy to improve your diet if you take it one step, one choice at a time. Start by choosing one challenge to work on, come up with a solution, and spend one week trying to correct it. After it's mastered, choose a second eating or beverage challenge, and then continue until you have a well-managed diet.

## ■ Nutrition and the Athlete

The food groups already presented form the foundation of the diet recommended for young athletes (Figure 10.6). Any of the plans presented serve as the nucleus for meals both in and out of athletic seasons. There is a vast leeway in the choice of foods within each of the food groups. Basic nutritional needs of athletes and nonathletes do not differ except in terms of calories.[27]

Total caloric needs vary with individual metabolism and physical activity. An intake of 2000 calories each day should be the bare minimum allowed for an athlete involved in a vigorous training program. The number of calories a young male athlete expends in serious training may range as high as 4000–6000 calories per day. Calorie intake that exceeds expenditure for basal body functions, for physical activity, and for growth of lean body mass, however, will still form body fat, so pay attention to your training diet.

A pre-game meal should:

- Support blood sugar levels to avoid hunger sensations.
- Leave the stomach and upper bowel empty at the time of competition.
- Provide maximum hydration.
- Minimize stomach upset; promote maximum performance.
- Provide a psychological edge by including foods the athlete likes and believes will make him or her win.

*Carbohydrates* in the diet will support blood sugar and provide glycogen stores to maintain these levels. Glycogen, the storage form of carbohydrate, seems to be the quickest and most efficient source of energy.

Good choices of high-carbohydrate foods are:

| | | |
|---|---|---|
| apples | cheese pizza | orange sherbet |
| applesauce | egg noodles | pancakes |
| bagels | graham crackers | (enriched) |
| baked potatoes | hard rolls | pears |
| baking powder | macaroni and | spaghetti |
| biscuits | cheese | sponge cake |
| bananas | mashed potatoes | sweet potatoes |
| boiled potatoes | oatmeal | waffles |
| bread (white, | oranges and | |
| whole wheat) | orange juice | |

Carbohydrates are digested more rapidly than protein and fat. A breakfast of toast and jam, cereal with low-fat milk, and fruit or juice will leave the stomach much sooner than a meal of eggs with steak, sausage, or bacon.

Optimum hydration is important to athletes, especially those involved in endurance events, such as long-distance swimming and running. The immediate pre-game diet should consist of two to three glasses of some beverage, with no fewer than eight full glasses each 24 hours.

Whole milk is not recommended because of its high fat content. Caffeine also should be avoided because it may increase nervous tension and agitation before the contest. Noncarbonated fruit drinks are generally good choices.

Athletes should avoid concentrated sources of simple sugar such as glucose tablets and undiluted honey, as they can cause gas distention and discomfort. Also, bulky foods high in fiber or cellulose are not good choices before an event.

Energy gels (highly concentrated carbohydrates) claim to quickly replace glycogen, the body's carbohydrate stores. Leading health/fitness professionals have stated:

> While gels may give endurance athletes an extra boost, most athletes can ensure they have adequate glycogen stores by eating foods rich in carbohydrates before and following exercise.[28]

Energy gels are best suited to endurance athletes who participate in aerobic exercise for more than 1½ to 2 hours . . . and they must have access to water to take them.[29]

Athletes should avoid heavily salted foods on the day of competition, because these can cause water retention, which decreases athletic performance.

The pre-game meal should be eaten 3 to 4 hours before the contest. For a highly demanding sport, a 1000-calorie meal is ideal. A 500-calorie meal can suffice for a sport that requires lower energy.

Athletes must be prepared physically to meet the special demands on their bodies. The starting block is sound nutrition knowledge, and practice. If you sacrifice physical excellence to an inefficient or harmful diet, reduced strength and endurance and a poor performance will be the result.

> *Basic nutritional needs of athletes and nonathletes do not differ except in terms of calories.*

## ■ Dietary Guidelines for Americans

Food alone cannot make a person healthy, but good eating habits based on moderation and variety can help keep a person healthy and even improve health. The following guidelines suggested for most Americans, developed by the U.S. Department of Agriculture, Human Nutrition Information Service, are printed in more detail in the eight-pamphlet series entitled, *Dietary Guidelines for Americans.*[30] In brief, most Americans need to pay more attention to the following guidelines.

**Eat a variety of foods.** No single food supplies all the essential nutrients in the amounts you need. The greater the variety, the less likely you are to develop either a deficiency or an excess of any single nutrient.

**Maintain healthy weight.** If you are too fat or too thin, your chances of developing health problems (for example, high blood pressure, diabetes, heart disease, certain cancers) increase. There is no one plan for maintaining healthy weight. If your concern is to lose fat weight, increase your physical activity, eat slowly, eat less fat and fatty foods, eat less sugar and sweets, avoid too much alcohol, don't skip meals, and use up more calories than you take in. (Weight management is discussed in more detail in Chapter 11.)

**Choose a diet low in fat, and cholesterol.** If you have a high blood cholesterol level, you have a greater chance of incurring a heart attack. A population such as that in the United States, with diets high in saturated fats and cholesterol, tend to produce high blood cholesterol levels.

*Cholesterol* is a necessary constituent of body tissues. When the circulating amount in the blood is higher than 200 milligrams (mg) (mild risk) or higher than 240 mg (high risk), it can cause early atherosclerosis. Atherosclerosis is a process of fatty build-up in the walls of the blood vessels, eventually leading to narrowing of the arteries and poor circulation. Cholesterol is one of the three major risk factors for coronary heart attack. (The other two are high blood pressure and cigarette smoking.)

*High-density lipoproteins (HDL),* also called "good cholesterol," coat the inside of the artery walls, providing a protective layer of grease to prevent fatty deposits from building up. They also serve as scavengers by actually *helping* dissolve fatty deposits when they do occur. A high amount in the blood indicates protection and a decrease in heart attack risk. Certain people genetically have higher amounts. HDL also can be increased by weight loss and by regular aerobic exercise. A very low level in the blood indicates serious risk for heart attack.

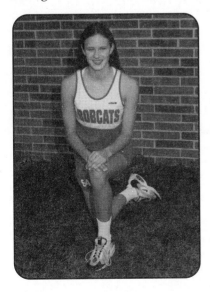

**Figure 10.6**
Nutrition and the athlete.

*Low-density lipoproteins (LDL)* are responsive to dietary habits and form dangerous deposits on the walls of blood vessels, are the primary culprits in clogged arteries and atherosclerosis, and place a person at high risk for heart attack. If cholesterol and HDL values are borderline, LDL values may decide the risk.

*Risk ratio* is a calculated value (total cholesterol divided by your HDL value) that most experts use to predict an individual's risk of heart attack in coming years. Having a high HDL cholesterol value and low LDL cholesterol value reduces the risk.

Cholesterol is measured by a simple blood test that shows milligrams (mg) of total cholesterol (HDL, LDL, and VLDL) per deciliter (dl) of blood.

If your blood lipid values are high and indicate increased risk for heart disease, you may benefit from improving your diet, increasing your exercise, or counseling concerning both.

*Triglycerides* (a type of fat) are diet-related and usually are not involved in the atherosclerosis process. High values occur in certain fat metabolism disorders and in diabetes.

Controversy surrounds recommendations for healthy Americans. For the U. S. population as a whole, however, reducing the intake of total fat, saturated fat, and cholesterol is sensible. Therefore:

■ Choose lean meats, fish, poultry, dry beans, and peas as your protein sources.

■ Moderate your intake of eggs and organ meats (such as liver).

■ Limit your intake of butter, cream, hydrogenated margarines, shortenings, coconut oil, and foods made from those products.

■ Trim excess fat from meats.

■ Broil, bake, and boil rather than fry.

■ Read food labels carefully to determine amounts and types of fat and cholesterol in foods.

■ Consume 300 mg/day (or less) of cholesterol.

■ Limit fat to 30% or less of total daily calories. To determine the *percentage* of calories that comes from fat in a product. Remember first that 1 gram of fat equals 9 calories. Multiply the grams of fat in a serving, times 9 calories. The result equals the number of *calories* from fat in one serving. Divide the fat calories in a serving by the total calories in a serving to determine the percentage of calories that comes from fat for one serving.

For example, if a chili label reads: "1 cup serving = 200 calories, fat 10g, carbohydrate 5g, sodium

980mg," then 1 cup of chili has 10 grams of fat. To figure the percentage of calories that comes from fat:

10g fat × 9 calories per gram =
90 calories from fat in 1 cup serving

90 fat calories ÷ 200 total calories =
45% of the calories in 1 cup of chili come from fat.[31]

**Choose a diet with plenty of vegetables, fruits, and grain products.** The major sources of energy in the average U. S. diet are carbohydrates and fats. Carbohydrates have an advantage over fats: They contain less than half the number of calories per ounce than fats.

Complex carbohydrate foods are better than simple carbohydrates. Simple carbohydrates (sugars) provide calories for energy but little else in the way of nutrients. Complex carbohydrates (beans, nuts, fruits, whole-grain breads) contain many essential nutrients plus calories for energy.

Increasing your consumption of certain complex carbohydrates also can increase dietary fiber, which tends to reduce the symptoms of chronic constipation, diverticulosis, and some types of irritable bowel. Diets low in fiber content also might increase the risk of developing cancer of the colon. Eating fruits, vegetables, and whole-grain breads and cereals will provide adequate fiber in the diet. Set a goal to increase dietary fiber to 20–30 grams per day.

**Use sugars in moderation.** The major hazard from eating too much sugar is tooth decay. The risk increases the more frequently you eat sugar and sweets, especially between meals, if you eat foods that stick to the teeth (sticky candy, dates), and if you consume soft drinks throughout the day.

■ Use less of all sugars (white, brown, raw, honey, and syrups).

■ Select fresh fruit or fruit canned without heavy syrup.

■ Read food labels for sugar information: If sucrose, glucose, maltose, dextrose, lactose, fructose, or syrup is listed as one of the first ingredients, the product has a lot of sugar.

To determine how many *teaspoons of sugar* a product contains, divide the grams in a serving by 5 (since there are 5 grams of sugar in 1 teaspoon).

For example, if a cereal box label reads:
"1-cup serving = 140 calories,
carbohydrates/starch 10g, sucrose 15g, fiber 1gm,"
then 1 cup of cereal contains 15 grams of sucrose;

and
15 grams of sucrose ÷ 5 grams of sugar per teaspoon =
3 teaspoons of simple sugar in 1 cup of cereal.

Products are healthier when sucrose (simple sugar) amounts are low.[32]

**Use salt and sodium only in moderation.** The major hazard posed by excessive sodium is its effect on blood pressure. In populations where high-sodium intake is common, high blood pressure is also common. In populations with low-sodium intake, high blood pressure is rare. Establish preventive measures, such as the following:

▪ Eliminate all salt use at the table.

▪ Cook with little or no salt.

▪ Select foods that are low in sodium content.

The dietary goal for sodium intake is approximately 2400 mg/day.

**If you drink alcoholic beverages, do so in moderation.** Alcoholic beverages tend to be high in calories and low in other nutrients. Heavy drinkers may lose their appetite for foods that contain essential nutrients. Vitamin and mineral deficiencies occur commonly in heavy drinkers because of poor nutrient intake and because alcohol alters absorption and use of some essential nutrients.

Although one or two drinks daily seem to cause no harm in adults, even moderate drinkers should remember that alcohol is a high-calorie, low-nutrient food. If you wish to achieve or maintain ideal weight, alcohol intake must be well monitored.

Women should consume no more than one drink a day, and men, no more than two drinks a day.

Research indicates that women have higher blood alcohol levels than men after having one drink. This is because women have less activity of an enzyme that helps metabolize alcohol in the body. Thus, women are more vulnerable to the acute and chronic complications of alcoholism.

*Count a drink as:*

▪ 12 fluid ounces of regular or light beer

▪ 5 fluid ounces of table wine

▪ 3½ fluid ounces of dessert wine

▪ 7 fluid ounces of light wine

▪ 1½ fluid ounces of gin, rum, whiskey (80 proof)

▪ 1 mixed drink.[33]

## SUMMARY

Better or best nutrition choices can be made by following the various guidelines mentioned in this chapter.

If you know little about human physiology — how your vital processes work — it's best not to resort to chance or whatever nutritional guidelines you encounter. An abundance of scientifically based, easy-to-read literature explains how to balance the needed nutrients. Select guidelines developed by well-established medical and fitness sources, such as those referred to in this chapter rather than those from your favorite movie and television stars or the supermarket trade magazines.

---

### Food and Beverage Intake Diary for One Day/Week

**Instructions:** Enjoy recording your food and beverage intake, one day at a time, for at least one week in your Fitness Journal. It will require just a moment's reflection as you identify the points listed. After one week, ask yourself: How do my choices measure up to the standards established for a balanced diet, with special attention to selecting nutrient-dense foods?

▪ Place a checkmark next to each nutrient-dense food choice you made, on the left, before each food/beverage entry.

▪ Identify the nutrient density rating for each food (4-star/3-star, etc.).

▪ Comment regarding the social and emotional aspects of your eating patterns.

▪ Practice the feeling sense and rate 0–10 how "empty"/"full" you feel before, during, and after your meals or snacks.

▪ Set a goal to improve one aspect of your diet or eating actions that need the most attention.

| Date: | *Nutrient Density | Name of Food | Food Groups: Mi/Me/V/F/B/SF | How Much | With Whom | | | Where | Eating Dial | | | Why | | | | | | | How Long (Number of Minutes) | Other Activity While Eating |
|---|---|---|---|---|---|---|---|---|---|---|---|---|---|---|---|---|---|---|---|---|
| | | | | | Alone | Family | Friends | | Before | During | After | Worried | Bored | Depressed | Tired | Social | Hungry | Other: | | |
| BREAKFAST | | | | | | | | | | | | | | | | | | | | |
| SNACK | | | | | | | | | | | | | | | | | | | | |
| LUNCH | | | | | | | | | | | | | | | | | | | | |
| SNACK | | | | | | | | | | | | | | | | | | | | |
| DINNER | | | | | | | | | | | | | | | | | | | | |
| SNACK | | | | | | | | | | | | | | | | | | | | |

## EXERCISE 10.1 Considerations for Vegetarian Meal Planning

**1** Identify the group(s) you're choosing to eat in an alternative way (meat group, milk group, meat and milk groups, fats/oils/sweets group) and the reason for each choice:

I am *alternatively* eating the: \_\_\_\_Meat Group
\_\_\_\_ Milk Group     \_\_\_\_Both Meat and Milk Group
\_\_\_\_ Fats, Oils, and Sweets Group.

**My reasons for this choice:** _____

**Here are six eating style definitions,** * **including each plan's name and the main food choices eaten. Check (✔) the plan you're choosing to eat:**

\_\_\_\_ *Animal/Meat-Based Diet:* beef, pork, chicken, turkey, fish, eggs, and dairy products

\_\_\_\_ *Plant-Based Diet:* fruits, vegetables, grains, legumes, seeds, and nuts

\_\_\_\_ *Vegetarian Diet:* plant-based diet that may include seafood, fish, eggs, or dairy products

\_\_\_\_ *Lacto-Ovo Vegetarian Diet:* plant-based diet plus eggs and dairy products

\_\_\_\_ *Lacto-Vegetarian Diet:* plant-based diet plus dairy products

\_\_\_\_ *Vegan (VEE-gun) Diet:* plant-based diet only (excludes all animal foods, meat, poultry, fish, eggs, and dairy products)

*From Tammy Kime-Sheets, author of original teaching tool entitled, *How To Eat Without The Meat,* in section "Cut The Animal Fat," p. 2, distributed to clients at Nutritional Wellness seminars and workshops in greater Toledo, OH area, 1996–1998.

**2** Do you understand *what the required nutrients and their functions are* **(that are provided in each group), that have to be considered and replaced by other forms of alternative food choices (that, likewise, can provide those required nutrients)?**

\_\_\_\_ **Yes. If your answer is** \_\_\_\_ **No:**

Especially consider your needs for all of the following essential nutrients and the functions each performs to keep you healthy: amino acids (ensuring adequate nitrogen retention); calcium; iron; linolenic acid; vitamin $B_{12}$; Vitamin D; zinc. Identify *naturally occurring foods* (not *manufactured* pills/potions/products) that you enjoy eating and drinking and an accompanying serving size you'll eat that provides each nutrient involved in your new plan.

| Nutrient | Foods I Enjoy That Provide This | A Serving Size Equals |
|---|---|---|
| Essential amino acids | _____ | _____ |
| Calcium | _____ | _____ |
| Iron | _____ | _____ |
| Linolenic acid | _____ | _____ |
| Vitamin $B_{12}$ | _____ | _____ |
| Vitamin D | _____ | _____ |
| Zinc | _____ | _____ |

This information is fully detailed on the Internet Web site of *The Vegetarian Resource Group* at **http://www.vrg.org/** and can provide you with valuable assistance in your meal planning for vegetarian eating.

**3** Does this new choice of eating plan fulfill *your* physical, social, emotional, spiritual, intellectual, and talent expression needs?

Answer these questions:

**Physical:** Will my food and beverage choices provide for all of my needs regarding basal metabolism, growth, repair, and energy? _____

(We usually find out the answer to this question when the *lack* shows up and we don't have enough nutrients present to provide needed energy/proper growth/ability to repair in a timely fashion/or when illness and disease take over.)

Do I eat a variety of food *colors (resembling a rainbow) and crunches** that provides naturally for these four needs? \_\_\_\_

**Social:** Can I *easily* eat my plan around family and friends, and *enjoy* all of my choices in their presence? _____

**Emotional:** Does my eating plan \_\_\_\_ *predominantly* include \_\_\_\_ *occasionally* include \_\_\_\_ *never* include "comfort" food I may choose to eat? (Comfort food is usually characterized as having a soft, mushy texture and is usually white, creamy, beige, or brown in color.) Are my eating choices primarily focused \_\_\_\_ *toward* promoting my best health or \_\_\_\_ *away from* experiencing illness and disease?

**Spiritual/Philosophical:** Does the eating plan I'm choosing to follow include a belief that "nature" can supply all the essential nutrients (from naturally existing sources), or must I rely on self-prescribed supplementation using *manufactured* pills, potions, and products to obtain all of the necessary nutrients I need to stay healthy?

\_\_\_\_ All from nature.

\_\_\_\_ Inadequate, so I must self-supplement to have all of the required nutrients I need.

**Intellectual:** Would my combined choices fulfill the eating guidelines established by the federal government, the American Dietetics Association, a local registered dietitian or licensed nutritionist, and/or my family physician?

\_\_\_\_ Yes, from any of these sources.

\_\_\_\_ No, not from any of these sources. The source for guidelines I choose to follow is:

_____

**Talent Expression:** If I am an athlete, is my eating plan providing all of the nutrients I need to stay well, grow, and repair, in addition to the increased energy and fluid replacement needs I have?

\_\_\_\_ Yes      \_\_\_\_ No

(Athletes in training must adjust to their increased energy needs by eating significantly more servings of the carbohydrate foods and replace the loss of fluids by consuming more water or other appropriate fluids.)

*From Tammy Kime-Sheets, *How To Eat Without The Meat,* in section "Lifestyle Profile of Nutrition Choice, You Are How You Eat," 1996–1998.

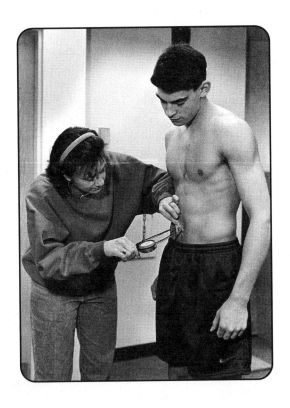

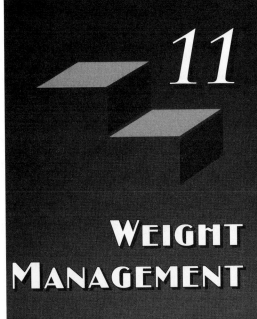

# 11

# WEIGHT MANAGEMENT

Your body is composed of two types of weight: lean weight and fat weight (also called lean body mass or fat-free mass, and fat mass). Lean weight is composed primarily of bones, muscles, internal organs, and body fluids. Your lean weight begins to weigh less after maturity when you stop growing at a certain steady pace every year. Fat weight is stored energy and protection for present and future use. The amount of each type of weight you carry is important to know so you can understand what is best for the health of your heart and lungs (cardiovascular and respiratory systems).

## Body Composition

Body fat can be classified as either essential fat or storage fat. *Essential fat* is needed for normal physiological functions. Without it, your health begins to deteriorate. This essential fat constitutes about 3% of the total fat in men and 10%–12% in women. The percentage is higher in women because it includes gender-related fat such as that found in the breast tissue, the uterus, and other gender-related areas.

*Storage fat* is the fat stored in adipose tissue, mostly beneath the skin (subcutaneous fat) and around major organs in the body. This fat serves three basic functions:

1. As an insulator to retain body heat
2. As energy substrate for metabolism
3. As padding against physical trauma to the body.

119

The amount of storage fat does not differ between men and women except that men tend to store fat around the waist and women more so around the hips and thighs.[1]

Each person can "wear" a certain percentage of fat to maintain ideal cardiovascular and respiratory efficiency and minimize the risk factors associated with heart disease. Perhaps you are wearing less than a recommended percentage of fat than is listed. This doesn't matter unless you are malnourishing yourself or you wish to look heavier cosmetically. A number of people don't wear the recommended percentages. For example, endurance athletes such as marathon runners and Olympic gymnasts carry much less fat. They burn it off and don't carry the excess. They usually eat right to provide the necessary nutrients and energy and thus display a firm, trim, toned look, yet they stay well.

In contrast are individuals who have the "starvation disease" anorexia nervosa. They, too, carry less than the suggested recommended percentage of body fat, but they do this by also eliminating their lean weight. They desire a trim look but go about it in a way that is against all physiological principles of proper weight loss. To them, weight loss means dropping pounds to be slim at all cost, no matter what kind of weight it is, fat or lean. This is an extremely detrimental way to lose weight. The concept of healthy slimness and unhealthy slimness is presented later in the chapter.

## Determining Your Recommended Weight

A recommended weight cannot be determined just by looking at someone. Therefore, an assessment determining an individual's body composition must be done. This includes calculating, as precisely as possible, one's body fat percentage in relation to one's lean weight mass. Knowing these values provides for an estimate to be made regarding an individual's "best" or recommended weight.

Two methods for determining your recommended weight (and the accompanying health risks from not maintaining that weight) are presented or referenced in this chapter:

1. *Measuring Skinfold Thickness.* This method is initially performed by a well-trained fitness professional using precision laboratory instruments, followed by each student using the number values received, to figure individual results. The formula to figure this method is provided in this chapter.

2. *Body Mass Index (BMI) Calculation.* This method can be easily calculated by the student, using a computer that has Internet capabilities, and a Web site accepted by the instructor. (With most of these sites, having access to a color printer will greatly enhance the visual learning presented!) A requirement to start this calculation is having a recent and accurate measurement of your weight (in pounds) and your height (in inches).

The BMI calculation procedure and all the necessary accompanying research (health risks related to the index value you are assigned), procedures to follow (properly measuring your height and weight to provide accuracy in your results), and suggestions to consider (eating and exercising to attain your recommended weight) are provided on several professionally rated sites[2] listed here.[3] Before beginning, review each site, including any your instructor may add to this list:

■ Shape Up America! — http://www.shapeup. org/sua/ *(Body Mass Index)*

■ Ask The Dietitian[sm] — www.dietitian.com/ibw/ ibw.html *(Healthy Body Calculator[sm])*

■ American Medical Association — http://www. ama.assn.org *(General Health/Interactive Health sections).*

Both of these methods approach the topic of determining one's recommended weight from a different perspective, and both have advantages and disadvantages. Therefore, it is suggested that students become aware of how *both* methods are calculated to obtain a recommended weight.

### Measuring Skinfold Thickness

The skinfold thickness measurement technique can determine whether an individual is at recommended weight, or is underweight, overweight (overfat), or obese, and then quantify exactly by how much. Specific goals then can be set to obtain, or maintain, recommended weight. Because of the relative accuracy, availability of equipment, and ease of use in a fitness class setting, measuring skinfold thickness is currently the most frequently used technique with this population. It has also been recorded as a more

*Body composition can be assessed by measuring skinfold thickness to determine your percentage of body fat and lean weight mass. With that information, an estimated recommended body weight can be established that is best for your cardiovascular and respiratory health.*

accurate method for certain populations to use, than is the Body Mass Index (BMI) Calculation referenced on page 118.

Assessment of body composition using skinfold thickness is based on the principle that approximately half of the body's fatty tissue is deposited directly beneath the skin. If this tissue is estimated validly and reliably, it can produce a good indication of percent body fat.

This test is done with the aid of a precision instrument called a *skinfold caliper*. Three specific sites must be measured with the calipers and then added together to reflect the total percentage of fat. These measurements may vary slightly on the same subject when they are taken by different professionals. Therefore, pre- and post-measurements preferably should be taken by the same technician.

Using the three-site skinfold testing, the procedure for assessing percent body fat follows:

1. Specific anatomical sites are tested. For men, these are the chest, abdomen, and thigh (Figure 11.1). For women, the suprailium, thigh, and triceps areas are tested (Figure 11.2). All measurements should be taken on the right side of the body with the subject standing.

2. The technician conducts the measurements by grasping a thickness of skin in the key locations just mentioned, with a thumb and forefinger, and pulling the fold slightly away from the muscular tissue. The calipers are held perpendicular to the fold, and the measurement is taken ½" below the finger hold. Each site is measured three times, and the values are read to the nearest .1 to .5 mm. The average of the two closest readings is recorded as your final value. The readings are taken in close succession to avoid excessive compression of the skinfold. Releasing and regrabbing the skinfold is required between readings.

3. When doing pre- and post-assessments, the measurement should be conducted at the same time of day. The best time is early in the morning to avoid hydration changes resulting from activity or exercise.

Record your findings in Figure 11.3. The percent fat is obtained by adding all three skinfold measurements and looking up the respective values on Table 11.1 for women, Table 11.2 for men under 40, and Table 11.3 for men over 40.

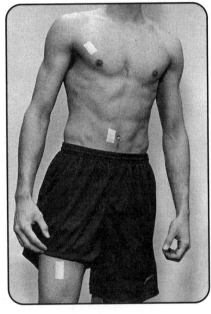

**Figure 11.1**
Anatomical sites for skinfold testing of men: chest, abdomen, and thigh.

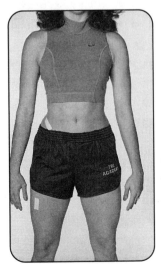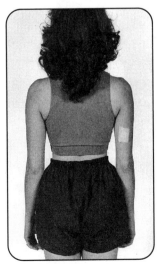

**Figure 11.2** Anatomical sites for skinfold testing of women: suprailium and thigh; triceps.

**TABLE 11.1  Percent Fat Estimates for Women Calculated from Triceps, Suprailium, and Thigh Skinfold Thickness**

| Sum of 3 Skin-folds | Under 22 | 23 to 27 | 28 to 32 | 33 to 37 | 38 to 42 | 43 to 47 | 48 to 52 | 53 to 57 | Over 58 |
|---|---|---|---|---|---|---|---|---|---|
| 23-25 | 9.7 | 9.9 | 10.2 | 10.4 | 10.7 | 10.9 | 11.2 | 11.4 | 11.7 |
| 26-28 | 11.0 | 11.2 | 11.5 | 11.7 | 12.0 | 12.3 | 12.5 | 12.7 | 13.0 |
| 29-31 | 12.3 | 12.5 | 12.8 | 13.0 | 13.3 | 13.5 | 13.8 | 14.0 | 14.3 |
| 32-34 | 13.6 | 13.8 | 14.0 | 14.3 | 14.5 | 14.8 | 15.0 | 15.3 | 15.5 |
| 35-37 | 14.8 | 15.0 | 15.3 | 15.5 | 15.8 | 16.0 | 16.3 | 16.5 | 16.8 |
| 38-40 | 16.0 | 16.3 | 16.5 | 16.7 | 17.0 | 17.2 | 17.5 | 17.7 | 18.0 |
| 41-43 | 17.2 | 17.4 | 17.7 | 17.9 | 18.2 | 18.4 | 18.7 | 18.9 | 19.2 |
| 44-46 | 18.3 | 18.6 | 18.8 | 19.1 | 19.3 | 19.6 | 19.8 | 20.1 | 20.3 |
| 47-49 | 19.5 | 19.7 | 20.0 | 20.2 | 20.5 | 20.7 | 21.0 | 21.2 | 21.5 |
| 50-52 | 20.6 | 20.8 | 21.1 | 21.3 | 21.6 | 21.8 | 22.1 | 22.3 | 22.6 |
| 53-55 | 21.7 | 21.9 | 22.1 | 22.4 | 22.6 | 22.9 | 23.1 | 23.4 | 23.6 |
| 56-58 | 22.7 | 23.0 | 23.2 | 23.4 | 23.7 | 23.9 | 24.2 | 24.4 | 24.7 |
| 59-61 | 23.7 | 24.0 | 24.2 | 24.5 | 24.7 | 25.0 | 25.2 | 25.5 | 25.7 |
| 62-64 | 24.7 | 25.0 | 25.2 | 25.5 | 25.7 | 26.0 | 26.2 | 26.4 | 26.7 |
| 65-67 | 25.7 | 25.9 | 26.2 | 26.4 | 26.7 | 26.9 | 27.2 | 27.4 | 27.7 |
| 68-70 | 26.6 | 26.9 | 27.1 | 27.4 | 27.6 | 27.9 | 28.1 | 28.4 | 28.6 |
| 71-73 | 27.5 | 27.8 | 28.0 | 28.3 | 28.5 | 28.8 | 29.0 | 29.3 | 29.5 |
| 74-76 | 28.4 | 28.7 | 28.9 | 29.2 | 29.4 | 29.7 | 29.9 | 30.2 | 30.4 |
| 77-79 | 29.3 | 29.5 | 29.8 | 30.0 | 30.3 | 30.5 | 30.8 | 31.0 | 31.3 |
| 80-82 | 30.1 | 30.4 | 30.6 | 30.9 | 31.1 | 31.4 | 31.6 | 31.9 | 32.1 |
| 83-85 | 30.9 | 31.2 | 31.4 | 31.7 | 31.9 | 32.2 | 32.4 | 32.7 | 32.9 |
| 86-88 | 31.7 | 32.0 | 32.2 | 32.5 | 32.7 | 32.9 | 33.2 | 33.4 | 33.7 |
| 89-91 | 32.5 | 32.7 | 33.0 | 33.2 | 33.5 | 33.7 | 33.9 | 34.2 | 34.4 |
| 92-94 | 33.2 | 33.4 | 33.7 | 33.9 | 34.2 | 34.4 | 34.7 | 34.9 | 35.2 |
| 95-97 | 33.9 | 34.1 | 34.4 | 34.6 | 34.9 | 35.1 | 35.4 | 35.6 | 35.9 |
| 98-100 | 34.6 | 34.8 | 35.1 | 35.3 | 35.5 | 35.8 | 36.0 | 36.3 | 36.5 |
| 101-103 | 35.2 | 35.4 | 35.7 | 35.9 | 36.2 | 36.4 | 36.7 | 36.9 | 37.2 |
| 104-106 | 35.8 | 36.1 | 36.3 | 36.6 | 36.8 | 37.1 | 37.3 | 37.5 | 37.8 |
| 107-109 | 36.4 | 36.7 | 36.9 | 37.1 | 37.4 | 37.6 | 37.9 | 38.1 | 38.4 |
| 110-112 | 37.0 | 37.2 | 37.5 | 37.7 | 38.0 | 38.2 | 38.5 | 38.7 | 38.9 |
| 113-115 | 37.5 | 37.8 | 38.0 | 38.2 | 38.5 | 38.7 | 39.0 | 39.2 | 39.5 |
| 116-118 | 38.0 | 38.3 | 38.5 | 38.8 | 39.0 | 39.3 | 39.5 | 39.7 | 40.0 |
| 119-121 | 38.5 | 38.7 | 39.0 | 39.2 | 39.5 | 39.7 | 40.0 | 40.2 | 40.5 |
| 122-124 | 39.0 | 39.2 | 39.4 | 39.7 | 39.9 | 40.2 | 40.4 | 40.7 | 40.9 |
| 125-127 | 39.4 | 39.6 | 39.9 | 40.1 | 40.4 | 40.6 | 40.9 | 41.1 | 41.4 |
| 128-130 | 39.8 | 40.0 | 40.3 | 40.5 | 40.8 | 41.0 | 41.3 | 41.5 | 41.8 |

NOTE: Body density is calculated based on the generalized equation for predicting body density of women developed by A. S. Jackson, M. L. Pollock, and A. Ward. *Medicine and Science in Sports and Exercise* 12:175-182, 1980. Percent body fat is determined from the calculated body density using the Siri formula.

**TABLE 11.2  Percent Fat Estimates for Men Under 40 Calculated from Chest, Abdomen, and Thigh Skinfold Thickness**

| Sum of 3 Skin-folds | Under 19 | 20 to 22 | 23 to 25 | 26 to 28 | 29 to 31 | 32 to 34 | 35 to 37 | 38 to 40 |
|---|---|---|---|---|---|---|---|---|
| 8-10 | .9 | 1.3 | 1.6 | 2.0 | 2.3 | 2.7 | 3.0 | 3.3 |
| 11-13 | 1.9 | 2.3 | 2.6 | 3.0 | 3.3 | 3.7 | 4.0 | 4.3 |
| 14-16 | 2.9 | 3.3 | 3.6 | 3.9 | 4.3 | 4.6 | 5.0 | 5.3 |
| 17-19 | 3.9 | 4.2 | 4.6 | 4.9 | 5.3 | 5.6 | 6.0 | 6.3 |
| 20-22 | 4.8 | 5.2 | 5.5 | 5.9 | 6.2 | 6.6 | 6.9 | 7.3 |
| 23-25 | 5.8 | 6.2 | 6.5 | 6.8 | 7.2 | 7.5 | 7.9 | 8.2 |
| 26-28 | 6.8 | 7.1 | 7.5 | 7.8 | 8.1 | 8.5 | 8.8 | 9.2 |
| 29-31 | 7.7 | 8.0 | 8.4 | 8.7 | 9.1 | 9.4 | 9.8 | 10.1 |
| 32-34 | 8.6 | 9.0 | 9.3 | 9.7 | 10.0 | 10.4 | 10.7 | 11.1 |
| 35-37 | 9.5 | 9.9 | 10.2 | 10.6 | 10.9 | 11.3 | 11.6 | 12.0 |
| 38-40 | 10.5 | 10.8 | 11.2 | 11.5 | 11.8 | 12.2 | 12.5 | 12.9 |
| 41-43 | 11.4 | 11.7 | 12.1 | 12.4 | 12.7 | 13.1 | 13.4 | 13.8 |
| 44-46 | 12.2 | 12.6 | 12.9 | 13.3 | 13.6 | 14.0 | 14.3 | 14.7 |
| 47-49 | 13.1 | 13.5 | 13.8 | 14.2 | 14.5 | 14.9 | 15.2 | 15.5 |
| 50-52 | 14.0 | 14.3 | 14.7 | 15.0 | 15.4 | 15.7 | 16.1 | 16.4 |
| 53-55 | 14.8 | 15.2 | 15.5 | 15.9 | 16.2 | 16.6 | 16.9 | 17.3 |
| 56-58 | 15.7 | 16.0 | 16.4 | 16.7 | 17.1 | 17.4 | 17.8 | 18.1 |
| 59-61 | 16.5 | 16.9 | 17.2 | 17.6 | 17.9 | 18.3 | 18.6 | 19.0 |
| 62-64 | 17.4 | 17.7 | 18.1 | 18.4 | 18.8 | 19.1 | 19.4 | 19.8 |
| 65-67 | 18.2 | 18.5 | 18.9 | 19.2 | 19.6 | 19.9 | 20.3 | 20.6 |
| 68-70 | 19.0 | 19.3 | 19.7 | 20.0 | 20.4 | 20.7 | 21.1 | 21.4 |
| 71-73 | 19.8 | 20.1 | 20.5 | 20.8 | 21.2 | 21.5 | 21.9 | 22.2 |
| 74-76 | 20.6 | 20.9 | 21.3 | 21.6 | 22.0 | 22.2 | 22.7 | 23.0 |
| 77-79 | 21.4 | 21.7 | 22.1 | 22.4 | 22.8 | 23.1 | 23.4 | 23.8 |
| 80-82 | 22.1 | 22.5 | 22.8 | 23.2 | 23.5 | 23.9 | 24.2 | 24.6 |
| 83-85 | 22.9 | 23.2 | 23.6 | 23.9 | 24.3 | 24.6 | 25.0 | 25.3 |
| 86-88 | 23.6 | 24.0 | 24.3 | 24.7 | 25.0 | 25.4 | 25.7 | 26.1 |
| 89-91 | 24.4 | 24.7 | 25.1 | 25.4 | 25.8 | 26.1 | 26.5 | 26.8 |
| 92-94 | 25.1 | 25.5 | 25.8 | 26.2 | 26.5 | 26.9 | 27.2 | 27.5 |
| 95-97 | 25.8 | 26.2 | 26.5 | 26.9 | 27.2 | 27.6 | 27.9 | 28.3 |
| 98-100 | 26.6 | 26.9 | 27.3 | 27.6 | 27.9 | 28.3 | 28.6 | 29.0 |
| 101-103 | 27.3 | 27.6 | 28.0 | 28.3 | 28.6 | 29.0 | 29.3 | 29.7 |
| 104-106 | 27.9 | 28.3 | 28.6 | 29.0 | 29.3 | 29.7 | 30.0 | 30.4 |
| 107-109 | 28.6 | 29.0 | 29.3 | 29.7 | 30.0 | 30.4 | 30.7 | 31.1 |
| 110-112 | 29.3 | 29.6 | 30.0 | 30.3 | 30.7 | 31.0 | 31.4 | 31.7 |
| 113-115 | 30.0 | 30.3 | 30.7 | 31.0 | 31.3 | 31.7 | 32.0 | 32.4 |
| 116-118 | 30.6 | 31.0 | 31.3 | 31.6 | 32.0 | 32.3 | 32.7 | 33.0 |
| 119-121 | 31.3 | 31.6 | 32.0 | 32.3 | 32.6 | 33.0 | 33.3 | 33.7 |
| 122-124 | 31.9 | 32.2 | 32.6 | 32.9 | 33.3 | 33.6 | 34.0 | 34.3 |
| 125-127 | 32.5 | 32.9 | 33.2 | 33.5 | 33.9 | 34.2 | 34.6 | 34.9 |
| 128-130 | 33.1 | 33.5 | 33.8 | 34.2 | 34.5 | 34.9 | 35.2 | 35.5 |

NOTE: Body density is calculated based on the generalized equation for predicting body density of men developed by A. S. Jackson, M. L. Pollock. *British Journal of Nutrition* 40:497-504, 1978. Percent body fat is determined from the calculated body density using the Siri formula.

**TABLE 11.3 Percent Fat Estimates for Men Over 40 Calculated from Chest, Abdomen, and Thigh Skinfold Thickness**

| Sum of 3 Skin-folds | Age to the Last Year | | | | | | | |
|---|---|---|---|---|---|---|---|---|
| | 41 to 43 | 44 to 46 | 47 to 49 | 50 to 52 | 53 to 55 | 56 to 58 | 59 to 61 | Over 62 |
| 8-10 | 3.7 | 4.0 | 4.4 | 4.7 | 5.1 | 5.4 | 5.8 | 6.1 |
| 11-13 | 4.7 | 5.0 | 5.4 | 5.7 | 6.1 | 6.4 | 6.8 | 7.1 |
| 14-16 | 5.7 | 6.0 | 6.4 | 6.7 | 7.1 | 7.4 | 7.8 | 8.1 |
| 17-19 | 6.7 | 7.0 | 7.4 | 7.7 | 8.1 | 8.4 | 8.7 | 9.1 |
| 20-22 | 7.6 | 8.0 | 8.3 | 8.7 | 9.0 | 9.4 | 9.7 | 10.1 |
| 23-25 | 8.6 | 8.9 | 9.3 | 9.6 | 10.0 | 10.3 | 10.7 | 11.0 |
| 26-28 | 9.5 | 9.9 | 10.2 | 10.6 | 10.9 | 11.3 | 11.6 | 12.0 |
| 29-31 | 10.5 | 10.8 | 11.2 | 11.5 | 11.9 | 12.2 | 12.6 | 12.9 |
| 32-34 | 11.4 | 11.8 | 12.1 | 12.4 | 12.8 | 13.1 | 13.5 | 13.8 |
| 35-37 | 12.3 | 12.7 | 13.0 | 13.4 | 13.7 | 14.1 | 14.4 | 14.8 |
| 38-40 | 13.2 | 13.6 | 13.9 | 14.3 | 14.6 | 15.0 | 15.3 | 15.7 |
| 41-43 | 14.1 | 14.5 | 14.8 | 15.2 | 15.5 | 15.9 | 16.2 | 16.6 |
| 44-46 | 15.0 | 15.4 | 15.7 | 16.1 | 16.4 | 16.8 | 17.1 | 17.5 |
| 47-49 | 15.9 | 16.2 | 16.6 | 16.9 | 17.3 | 17.6 | 18.0 | 18.3 |
| 50-52 | 16.8 | 17.1 | 17.5 | 17.8 | 18.2 | 18.5 | 18.8 | 19.2 |
| 53-55 | 17.6 | 18.0 | 18.3 | 18.7 | 19.0 | 19.4 | 19.7 | 20.1 |
| 56-58 | 18.5 | 18.8 | 19.2 | 19.5 | 19.9 | 20.2 | 20.6 | 20.9 |
| 59-61 | 19.3 | 19.7 | 20.0 | 20.4 | 20.7 | 21.0 | 21.4 | 21.7 |
| 62-64 | 20.1 | 20.5 | 20.8 | 21.2 | 21.5 | 21.9 | 22.2 | 22.6 |
| 65-67 | 21.0 | 21.3 | 21.7 | 22.0 | 22.4 | 22.7 | 23.0 | 23.4 |
| 68-70 | 21.8 | 22.1 | 22.5 | 22.8 | 23.2 | 23.5 | 23.9 | 24.2 |
| 71-73 | 22.6 | 22.9 | 23.3 | 23.6 | 24.0 | 24.3 | 24.7 | 25.0 |
| 74-76 | 23.4 | 23.7 | 24.1 | 24.4 | 24.8 | 25.1 | 25.4 | 25.8 |
| 77-79 | 24.1 | 24.5 | 24.8 | 25.2 | 25.5 | 25.9 | 26.2 | 26.6 |
| 80-82 | 24.9 | 25.3 | 25.6 | 26.0 | 26.3 | 26.6 | 27.0 | 27.3 |
| 83-85 | 25.7 | 26.0 | 26.4 | 26.7 | 27.1 | 27.4 | 27.8 | 28.1 |
| 86-88 | 26.4 | 26.8 | 27.1 | 27.5 | 27.8 | 28.2 | 28.5 | 28.9 |
| 89-91 | 27.2 | 27.5 | 27.9 | 28.2 | 28.6 | 28.9 | 29.2 | 29.6 |
| 92-94 | 27.9 | 28.2 | 28.6 | 28.9 | 29.3 | 29.6 | 30.0 | 30.3 |
| 95-97 | 28.6 | 29.0 | 29.3 | 29.7 | 30.0 | 30.4 | 30.7 | 31.1 |
| 98-100 | 29.3 | 29.7 | 30.0 | 30.4 | 30.7 | 31.1 | 31.4 | 31.8 |
| 101-103 | 30.0 | 30.4 | 30.7 | 31.1 | 31.4 | 31.8 | 32.1 | 32.5 |
| 104-106 | 30.7 | 31.1 | 31.4 | 31.8 | 32.1 | 32.5 | 32.8 | 33.2 |
| 107-109 | 31.4 | 31.8 | 32.1 | 32.4 | 32.8 | 33.1 | 33.5 | 33.8 |
| 110-112 | 32.1 | 32.4 | 32.8 | 33.1 | 33.5 | 33.8 | 34.2 | 34.5 |
| 113-115 | 32.7 | 33.1 | 33.4 | 33.8 | 34.1 | 34.5 | 34.8 | 35.2 |
| 116-118 | 33.4 | 33.7 | 34.1 | 34.4 | 34.8 | 35.1 | 35.5 | 35.8 |
| 119-121 | 34.0 | 34.4 | 34.7 | 35.1 | 35.4 | 35.8 | 36.1 | 36.5 |
| 122-124 | 34.7 | 35.0 | 35.4 | 35.7 | 36.1 | 36.4 | 36.7 | 37.1 |
| 125-127 | 35.3 | 35.6 | 36.0 | 36.3 | 36.7 | 37.0 | 37.4 | 37.7 |
| 128-130 | 35.9 | 36.2 | 36.6 | 36.9 | 37.3 | 37.6 | 38.0 | 38.5 |

NOTE: Body density is calculated based on the generalized equation for predicting body density of men developed by A. S. Jackson, M. L. Pollock. *British Journal of Nutrition* 40:497-504, 1978. Percent body fat is determined from the calculated body density using the Siri formula.

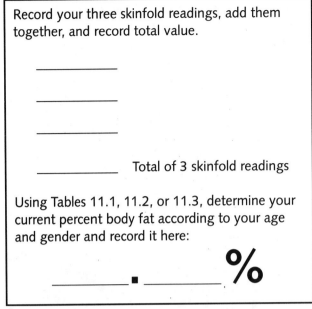

**Figure 11.3** Calculating Your Percent Body Fat

After finding out your percent body fat, you can determine your current body composition classification according to Table 11.4. In this table you will find the "health fitness" and the "high physical fitness" percent fat standards. For example, the recommended health fitness fat percentage for a 20-year-old female is 28% or less. The health fitness standard is established at the point where there seems to be no detriment to health in terms of percent body fat. A high physical fitness range for this same woman is between 18% and 23%.

My current classification label is:_____.

The high physical fitness standard does not mean that you cannot be somewhat below this number. As mentioned earlier, many highly trained athletes measurements are below the percentages set. The 3% essential fat for men and 12% for women are the lower limits for people to maintain good health. Below these percentages, normal physiologic functions can be seriously impaired.

In addition, some experts point out that a little storage fat (over the essential fat) is better than none at all. As a result, the health and high fitness standards for percent fat in Table 11.4 are set higher than the minimum essential fat requirements, at a point conducive to optimal health and well-being. Also, because lean tissue decreases with age, one extra percentage point is allowed for every additional decade of life. To calculate your recommended body weight, see Figures 11.4 and 11.5.

**TABLE 11.4    Body Composition Classification According to Percent Body Fat**

## MEN

| Age | Excellent | Good | Moderate | Overweight | Obese |
|-----|-----------|------|----------|------------|-------|
| ≤19 | 12.0 | 12.1-17.0 | 17.1-22.0 | 22.1-27.0 | ≥27.1 |
| 20-29 | 13.0 | 13.1-18.0 | 18.1-23.0 | 23.1-28.0 | ≥28.1 |
| 30-39 | 14.0 | 14.1-19.0 | 19.1-24.0 | 24.1-29.0 | ≥29.1 |
| 40-49 | 15.0 | 15.1-20.0 | 20.1-25.0 | 25.1-30.0 | ≥30.1 |
| ≥50 | 16.0 | 16.1-21.5 | 21.1-26.0 | 26.1-31.0 | ≥31.1 |

## WOMEN

| Age | Excellent | Good | Moderate | Overweight | Obese |
|-----|-----------|------|----------|------------|-------|
| ≤19 | 17.0 | 17.1-22.0 | 22.1-27.0 | 27.1-32.0 | ≥32.1 |
| 20-29 | 18.0 | 18.1-23.0 | 23.1-28.0 | 28.1-33.0 | ≥33.1 |
| 30-39 | 19.0 | 19.1-24.0 | 24.1-29.0 | 29.1-34.0 | ≥34.1 |
| 40-49 | 20.0 | 20.1-25.0 | 25.1-30.0 | 30.1-35.0 | ≥35.1 |
| ≥50 | 21.0 | 21.1-26.5 | 26.1-31.0 | 31.1-36.0 | ≥36.1 |

■ "High physical fitness" standard

■ "Health fitness" standard

Source: *Principles & Labs for Physical Fitness & Wellness* by Werner W. K. Hoeger (Englewood, CO: Morton Publishing Company, 1994), p. 62.

Your recommended body weight is computed based on your choosing a "health" or a "high fitness" fat percentage for your respective age and gender. Your selection of a desired fat percentage should be based on:

■ your current percent body fat; and

■ your personal health-fitness goals and objectives.

Select your desired/recommended body fat percentage from Table 11.4 based on your goals and the "health" or "high fitness" standards given. Express this percentage in decimal form:

._____% (RFP) GOAL


TIME FRAME: _____

**Figure 11.4**  Goal Setting Challenge

## DETERMINING YOUR RECOMMENDED BODY WEIGHT

1. **Fat Weight:** Multiply your total body weight in pounds (BW) by the current percent fat (%F) you're carrying (see Tables 11.1, 11.2, and 11.3), expressing this percentage in decimal form. (BW × ._____ % F). This is your *fat weight* (FW), the actual number of pounds of fat you now carry.

2. **Lean Weight:** Subtract your fat weight (FW) from your total body weight (BW − FW). This is your current *lean weight* (LW).

3. Place your desired/**recommended fat percentage** (RFP) you selected here (see Goal Setting Challenge, Figure 11.4), expressing this percentage in decimal form:

4. **Recommended Weight:** To calculate your recommended weight, use the following formula: LW ÷ (1.0 − .RFP) = RW (Recommended Weight).

**GOAL:** Subtract your recommended body weight from your current weight (BW − RW). This tells you exactly how many pounds you'll goal-set to lose or gain. (Note: Positive numbers = Weight to *lose*. Negative numbers = weight to *gain*.)

### CALCULATE HERE:

$$\underline{\quad\quad} \times .\underline{\quad\quad} = \underline{\quad\quad}$$
(BW   ×   % F   =   FW)

$$\underline{\quad\quad} - \underline{\quad\quad} = \underline{\quad\quad}$$
(BW   −   FW   =   LW)

._____ % (RFP)

$$\underline{\quad\quad} \div (1.0 - .\underline{\quad\quad}) = \underline{\quad\quad}$$
LW         RFP      RW

$$\underline{\quad\quad} - RW = \underline{\quad\quad\quad\quad}$$
BW           Actual pounds I'm setting a goal to lose/gain.

---

**Example:** A 19-year-old-female who weighs 136 pounds and is 25% fat would like to know what her recommended weight should be, with a "desired"/recommended fat percentage of 17%, which is the "high physical fitness" standard.

| | |
|---|---|
| Sex: | female |
| Age: | 19 |
| BW: | 136 lbs |
| %F: | 25% (.25 in decimal form) |
| RFP: | 17% (.17 in decimal form) |

■ FW = BW × %F
FW = 136 × .25 = 34 lbs.

■ LW = BW − FW
LW = 136 − 34 = 102 lbs.

■ RFP: 17% (.17 in decimal form)

■ RW = LW ÷ (1.0 − .RFP)
RW = 102 ÷ (1.0 − .17)
RW = 102 ÷ (.83) = 122.9 lbs.*

*(Recommended Body Weight)

**GOAL:** To reach her recommended body weight, she'll set a goal to lose 13.1 pounds of fat weight (subtracting recommended body weight from her current weight (136 − 122.9 = 13.1).

### GOAL SET TIMEFRAME TO LOSE/GAIN WEIGHT:

_____ /
1 week

_____ /
1 month

_____ /
3 months

_____ /
6 months

_____ /
1 year

**Figure 11.5**   Determining your recommended body weight.

## ■ Achieving a Healthy Slimness

We seem to admit readily that a primary goal in taking fitness courses is to *appear* healthy and slim. We desire this goal because we can see directly when our body looks nice, lean, and toned; likewise, we can see directly when it looks out of shape and flabby. Many individuals, therefore, focus initially on a form of "fitness" or "being in shape" that they can readily see.

Your outer appearance, however, is not the entire, or even major, focus of a quality fitness program. You can live without well-toned muscles or a trim figure, but you can't live very long without a strong heart and lungs. Looking attractive and feeling good about your appearance are good ancillary goals (Figure 11.6). The key word, however, is *healthy* slimness. This will require developing a weight management program.

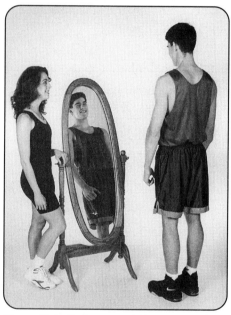

**Figure 11.6** Outer appearance, a secondary goal.

## ■ Principles of Weight Management

Weight management means controlling the amount of body fat in relation to the amount of lean tissue. Principles of weight management include:

1. *Weight maintenance* (keeping the same ratio of fat to amount of lean you're currently carrying).

2. *Weight gain* (almost always in terms of lean weight gain, not fat weight gain).

3. *Weight loss* (always in terms of loss of body fat).

## Weight Maintenance

Weight maintenance means that your current body composition of fat to lean is ideal for your best cardiovascular and respiratory health, and that you are pleased with how you look. You have enough strength to function well in your daily life of work and recreation, to whatever extreme that may encompass. To remain at this constant weight, your energy must be in balance:

calories in (eating) = calories out (exercise).

Calculate the calories for your weight maintenance on Figure 11.7. Because "calories out" declines with aging (the metabolism slows down and people are less active), a decline in "calories in" (eating less) must accompany the aging processes.

## Weight Gain

Weight gain almost always refers to gaining *lean* tissue, or thickening muscle fiber. When you want to look better cosmetically or to increase your strength for a sport or for daily needs, weight training is the type of activity in which to engage. If you are at an overfat weight, to *gain lean weight and lose extra body fat* simultaneously will require you to eat less

---

1. Record your present weight, in pounds.
2. Record your type of lifestyle. Number values are:

   12 = sedentary

   15 = active physically

   18 = pregnant/nursing

   20 = varsity athlete or physical laborer

3. Multiply (1) × (2).

This is your weight maintenance number, or the number of *calories per day you need to eat to stay at your current weight.*

　　_____　(1) weight

×　_____　(2) lifestyle
　　_____

　　_____　calories for weight
　　　　　　　maintenance

Source: *The Aerobic Way*, by Kenneth H. Cooper (New York: Evans & Co., 1977, p. 142.

**Figure 11.7** Calculating Weight Maintenance

while providing *more exercise* through weight training. Only if you are at a recommended weight or underfat weight should you accompany this weight-gain program with an increase in caloric intake.[4]

Weight gain, then, means increasing muscle mass, or thickening of muscle fibers. You do not gain more muscle cells; you thicken what you presently have.

## Weight Loss

Weight loss refers to purposefully losing *fat weight*, never lean weight. The weight lost, of course, can be both lean and fat, according to how you go about losing the weight. Before you spend your money on any unique new weight reduction plan, claim, product, device, or book, call your local Better Business Bureau. If you completely understand the principles of weight loss, you will be able to determine a product's or program's worth before you spend time, money, and energy on it. These principles are as follows.

1. *Fat weight is the only kind of weight to lose.* If a product or program claims to "get rid of excess body fluids," beware! Body fluids are not fat. Unnatural water retention, *edema*, is a condition to be monitored and treated by a doctor, not by self-prescribed procedures or products.

2. *If water weight (fluid) is lost by sweating during exercise, it will and should return in 24 hours* to maintain the body's chemical balance. The energy-producing (metabolic) processes perform best when all of the necessary components are present. Dropping water weight is not effective weight loss. It is part of the fat-free weight and is vital to continuous well-being. You can understand, then, why weighing yourself after a strenuous exercise session is an inaccurate time to weigh.

3. *Fat is metabolized more readily and efficiently by performing moderate-intensity exercise for a long time.* If you are able to work continuously at a moderate intensity (lower end of your training zone) for more than 30 minutes, you will tap into the most physiologically sound way to metabolize (burn off) unwanted body fat. You need to exercise for *more than 30 minutes at a time to make significant changes in the fat content of the body.*

    To maximize metabolism efficiency, increase one, two, or all three of the aerobic exercise criteria: *frequency*, *intensity*, and *time duration*. Refer to Chapters 1 and 2 for a review of what maximum levels of each can be safe for you to use.

Wearing rubber suits, transparent plastic wrap-around body parts, or heavy, long-sleeved sweats, pantyhose, or tights on hot days inhibits the free flow of sweat and does not allow it to perform its function of cooling. In hot and humid settings, wear as little as possible when performing fitness exercises. You cannot metabolize (burn up) fat faster by wearing more clothes.

4. *Fat burns off your body in a general way.* You can't "spot-reduce." Spot-reducing is perhaps the most prevalent misconception concerning fat weight loss. Many unscrupulous people are defrauding unsuspecting overfat Americans out of millions of dollars every year.

    By your genetic constitution, your body will use up its stored energy (fat) any way it is programmed to do. You cannot do 50 leg lifts a day and hope to reduce fat deposits in the area. You will shape up (thicken) the muscle fiber in the area, and toned muscles contain more of the enzymes involved in breaking down fat, but you do not burn off the fat there or at any specific location. As energy is needed, it is withdrawn first from the immediate sources, and when this is used up, randomly from more permanent storage. It then is converted to an immediate usable form. Thus, at first you may lose weight in places you don't necessarily wish to, such as your face or chest/breast area. With perseverance, however, you'll burn off the fat in problem areas, too.

5. *Loss of fat weight is accomplished most readily through a combined program of monitoring your food intake carefully and exercising aerobically.* When you monitor food intake (and eat less) and exercise (expend more calories or energy), you lose almost 100% fat. This is the only kind of weight you want to lose. Exercise speeds weight loss, by burning calories while you're working out and also by revitalizing your metabolism so you continue to burn calories more readily for the next few hours.

    Losing fat weight by simply eating less food is difficult. If you avoid exercise and severely restrict food intake only, the weight loss is not just fat. According to the way in which you have "dieted," your weight loss is approximately one-half to two-thirds fat loss and *one-third to one-half lean weight loss.* If your lifestyle and habits of eating and exercising don't change after you stop "dieting" and you gain back your lost weight, what you gain back is all fat. You are worse off because you lost both fat and lean tissue and regained only fat. Over a lifetime of yo-yo crash dieting, the entire body composition changes to your detriment.

You can *lose* fat weight in many ways. The only way to *keep* fat weight off is by following a regular exercise program.[5]

6. *Weight can be both gained or lost through an endurance exercise program.* You will be burning off fat for energy and building up muscle simultaneously. Therefore, if you do not see a change on the scale immediately, don't be disappointed.

7. *A light exercise program tends to increase appetite, and a strenuous exercise program decreases appetite.* After an endurance (aerobic) hour, the desire for food diminishes greatly. You will have time to carefully select or prepare what you know is good for you rather than ravenously grab that easy, high-calorie "no-star, sometimes" (see Chapter 10) food just sitting around.

8. *Eating less food is easier than exercising it off.* In most high-intensity fitness sessions, you will burn only about 300 calories. If you are seriously interested in losing extra fat weight, think twice about rewarding yourself with high-caloric treats afterward. Instead, replenish your water loss with noncaloric, yet quite filling, ice water.

9. *There is no such thing as a constipated endurance aerobic exerciser or athlete.* Regular, rhythmic stimulation of the entire digestion and elimination processes is one of the side benefits of aerobic exercise.

10. *The body's energy balance determines whether a person gains or loses body fat.* Proper weight loss is the result of *taking in less caloric energy and expending more.*

## ■ Weight-Loss Strategies

The challenge involved in losing weight may involve the need for any of the following: (a) a better self-image, (b) a naturally slender eating strategy, (c) learning effective ways to become motivated and make decisions, (d) resolving a phobic response to childhood abuse, (e) learning better social skills, or (f) learning better coping skills.[6]

## "Naturally Slender" Eating

One of the main differences between naturally slender and overweight individuals is their mental images and self-talk concerning food. Overweight people usually construct *present-tense* pictures and self-talk. They see, smell, hear, experience food, and state internally, "Boy, am I hungry!" The result is that they eat immediately. They focus only on the moment, as they eat.

Naturally thin people usually do not have this present-tense strategy. They create *future-tense* pictures, self-talk, and feelings. They experience how they'll feel over time[7] (see Figure 11.8). Naturally slender people, as they approach a restaurant food bar or order from a menu, determine *ahead of time* how they choose to feel *when they are all finished eating.* This proactive, plan-ahead approach can be the difference between being naturally slender or being overweight for a lifetime.

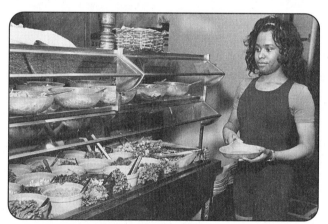

**Figure 11.8** Creating future-tense pictures, self-talk, and feelings before you select food.

## Control Panel With One Large Dial

A control panel with one large dial can be used as an eating strategy, to reflect how "empty" or "full" you feel:

— before you eat
— during the meal
— when you're done eating.

*Before you select,* you have to "go inside" where your hunger cues are. Predetermine how empty or full you are. Give that feeling a number from 0 to 10 and an accompanying label, as shown in Figure 11.9.

Then, when selecting and eating food, imagine your control panel and adjust it to how you feel currently, how you choose to feel during the eating process, and how you choose to feel when you're done eating and drinking. Add this feeling sense to the 1-day/week monitoring of your eating and beverage intake form found in Chapter 10, and record in your Fitness Journal.

## Caloric Intake and Use

Everything you eat or drink becomes *you* for either a short or a long time. You are what you eat and drink. The food nutrients you eat maintain basic body functions such as breathing, blood circulation, normal body temperature, and growth and repair of all tissue. These are related to fixed factors such as age, body size, and physiological state. Any kind of caloric intake your body doesn't use or doesn't eliminate through solid or liquid waste is kept and worn as body fat for future energy needs.

## Caloric Expenditure

Every moment of every day, no matter what activity you engage in, from sleeping to aerobic exercise, you are using up calories. *Caloric energy expenditure is influenced most by how physically active you are all* *day*. The body's basic needs are more or less fixed, but the amount of physical exertion is a personal decision.

How physically active your life is depends on your choices of profession and recreational activities. It depends upon a multitude of day-to-day choices: whether to walk to the local store or drive the car; use the stairs or elevator; rake the leaves or hire it done; go out for a bicycle ride after supper or watch a TV show. How physically active your life is depends as much on attitude as it does on opportunity.[8]

## Caloric Expenditures for Various Activities

How many calories you burn per minute during any activity depends upon two criteria:

1. *Intensity* (high-, medium-, or low-level work or exercise)
2. *Body weight.*

The higher the intensity, the more calories you burn per minute. For example, you expend more energy and calories running a mile than you do walking that mile. The more you weigh, the more

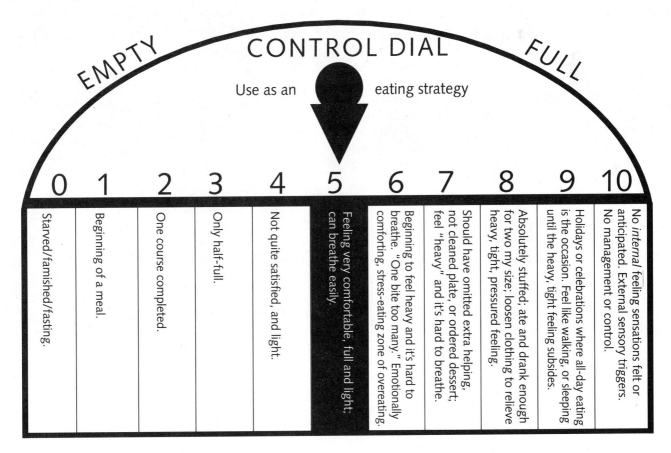

**Figure 11.9** Control Panel with One Large Dial.

calories per minute you will burn (just as full-size cars burn more fuel per mile than small, compact models).

## Caloric Intake Needed to Gain Lean Weight

To add 1 pound of body muscle requires 2500 calories. (This includes about 600 calories for the muscle and the extra energy needed for exercise to develop the muscle.) Thus, the daily caloric excess, over your maintenance number just figured, is 360.[9] You must be at or below your ideal weight to go on an excess calorie-eating program to gain muscle. You want to use your excess body fat first for your energy requirements.

*To gain 1 pound of muscle:*
2500 calories equivalent to 1 pound of muscle
÷ 7 days in a week
= 360 daily excess calories to eat over your
    maintenance intake number

Taking in more than 1000 calories per day over the number needed to maintain weight, however, is likely to result in weight gain as body fat even if you are exercising strenuously on a regular basis.[10]

## Caloric Intake Needed to Lose Body Fat

To lose more than 2 to 3 pounds of body fat per week is physiologically impossible.[11] Weight loss greater than this is in the form of water and lean body tissue. To drop unwanted extra body fat systematically, you need to drop 3500 calories a week, or 500 calories per day, to lose one pound of body fat per week.

*To lose 1 pound fat:*
3500 calories
÷ 7 days per week
= 500 calories a day fewer than your
    maintenance number

If you desire to drop more pounds per week but the total caloric intake would be less than 1200, you need to reestablish your goal to lose only 1 pound per week. You never want to eat fewer than 1200 calories per day. A daily diet of fewer than 1200 calories is likely to be deficient in needed nutrients for you to grow, repair, stay well, and have energy to perform daily tasks and leisure. Sometimes, on a one-to-one basis, a doctor will have a patient eat fewer than 1200 calories per day but will provide extensive guidelines and supplementation. This should be done *only* under the strict supervision of a doctor.

## SUMMARY

To maintain a specific weight, caloric input must equal caloric output. To gain or lose weight requires an imbalance of energy in your eating and exercising lifestyle habits.

To provide a continual means of self-discipline concerning your weight management:

- Assess your weight whenever your lean or fat weight has increased or decreased substantially.
- Get involved in programs that assist you in continuing to monitor your lifestyle habits.
- Enjoy the process of reviewing your time priorities and setting short- and long-range goals to achieve or maintain a recommended weight.

Educating yourself about how to manage your weight can be fascinating. It will help you understand how the human body works and how it does not work physiologically. You then can be alert to all of the false notions, especially regarding weight loss, that are rampant today. Equipped with accurate information, you can develop a program that will work for you for a lifetime!

# REFERENCES

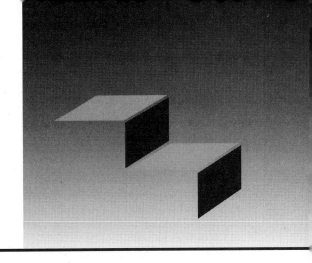

### ▬▬ Chapter 1

1. Ralph Paffenbarger et al., *New England Journal of Medicine*, 314: 10, (March 6, 1986).
2. Kenneth H. Cooper, *Run Dick, Fun Jane* (Film). (Provo, UT: Brigham Young University, 1971).
3. Cooper, *The Aerobics Way* (New York: M. Evans and Co., 1977), p. 10.
4. National Vital Statistics Division, Center for Health Statistics, Rockville, MD, 1988.
5. American College of Sports Medicine, "Position Stand, The Recommended Quality and Quantity of Exercise for Developing and Maintaining Cardiorespiratory and Muscular Fitness in Healthy Adults," *Medicine and Science in Sport Exercise*, 22:2 (1990), pp. 265-274.
6. Cooper, *Run Dick, Run Jane*.
7. Lenore R. Zohman et al., *The Cardiologists' Guide to Fitness and Health Through Exercise* (New York: Simon and Schuster, 1979), p. 72.
8. *Harvard Medical School Health Letter*, 10:6 (April 1985), p. 3.
9. *Harvard Medical School Health Letter*.
10. *Harvard Medical School Health Letter*.
11. ACSM Position Stand, 1990.
12. ACSM Position Stand.
13. American College of Sports Medicine, Resource Manual: Guidelines for Exercise Testing and Prescription, 3d edition (Baltimore: Williams & Wilkins, 1998).
14. ACSM's Resource Manual.
15. ACSM's Resource Manual.
16. G. A. V. Borg, "Psychophysical Bases of Perceived Exertion," *Medicine and Science in Sport and Exercise* 14 (1982). Also, Karen S. Mazzeo, *Aerobics, The Way To Fitness* (Englewood, CO: Morton Publishing, 1992), p. 18.
17. Charlotte A. Williams, "THR Versus RPE. The Debate Over Monitoring Exercise Intensity," *IDEA Today*, April 1991, p. 42.
18. Williams, p. 42.
19. *Surgeon General's Report*, Centers For Disease Control & Prevention (CDC) and the President's Council on Physical Fitness in Sports, Washgton, DC.

### ▬▬ Chapter 2

1. Kenneth H. Cooper, *Running Without Fear* (New York: M. Evans and Co., 1985), p. 128.
2. Cooper, p. 192.
3. Cooper, p. 197.
4. New York: M. Evans and Co. (1982), p. 141.
5. R. Cotton. Testing and Evaluation, in *Personal Trainer Manual: The Resource for Fitness Instructors* edited by M. Sudy (San Diego: American Council on Exercise, 1991), pp. 155-192.
6. L.A. Golding, C.R. Myers, & W. E. Sinning, *Y's Way to Physical Fitness*, 3d edition (Champaign, IL: Human Kinetics Publishers, 1989).
7. Werner W. K. Hoeger, *Principles & Labs for Physical Fitness & Wellness*. (Englewood, CO: Morton Publishing, 1991), pp. 133, 135.
8. Werner W. K. Hoeger, *Lifetime Physical Fitness and Wellness: A Personalized Program*. (Englewood, CO: Morton Publishing, 1986), p. 47.

### ▬▬ Chapter 3

1. Joan M. A. Price, "Stepping Basics," *IDEA Today*, November/December 1990. p. 57.
2. Len M. A. Kravitz, "The Safe Way To Step." *IDEA Today*, April 1991, pp. 47-50.
3. Sports Step, Inc. videotape accompanying The Step, *Introduction To Step Training*, Atlanta 1989.
4. Lynne Brick and David Essel videotape, *Pump N' Step* [videotape], 1991.
5. Lorna Francis, Peter Francis and Gin Miller, *Step-Reebok. The First Aerobic Training Workout with Muscle: Instructor Training Manual*. (Reebok International Ltd., 1990).
6. Lorna, p. 6.
7. M. S. Olson, et al., "Cardiorespiratory Responses to 'Aerobic' Bench Stepping Exercise in Females," *Medicine and Science in Sports and Exercise* (abstract), 23: 4 (April 1991), S27.
8. D. L. Blessing, et al., "The Energy Cost of Bench Stepping With and Without One and Two Pound Hand-Held Weights," *Medicine and Science in Sports and Exercise* (abstract), 23: 4 (April 1991), S28.
9. F. Goss, et al., "Energy Cost of Bench Stepping and Pumping Light Handweights in Trained Subjects," *Research Quarterly for Exercise and Sport*, 60: 4 (1989), pp. 369-372.
10. L. Calarco, et al., "The Metabolic Cost of Six Common Movement Patterns of Bench Step Aerobic Dance," *Medicine and Science in Sports and Exercise* (abstract), 23: 4 (April 1991), S140.

11. Ralph La Forge, "What the Latest Research Has to Say About STEP Exercise," *IDEA Today,* September, 1991, pp. 31-35.
12. D. Stanforth, et al., "The Effect of Bench Height and Rate of Stepping on the Metabolic Cost of Bench Stepping," *Medicine and Science in Sports and Exercise* (abstract), 23: 4 (April 1991), S143.
13. American College of Sports Medicine, "Position Statement on the Recommended Quantity and Quality of Exercise for Developing and Maintaining Cardiorespiratory and Muscular Fitness in Healthy Adults," *Medicine and Science in Sports and Exercise,* 22 (1990), pp. 265- 274.
14. M. S. Olson, et al., "The Physiological Effects of Bench/ Step Exercise," *Sports Medicine,* 3 (1996), pp. 164-175.
15. S. Woodby-Brown, K. Berg, and R. W. Latin, "Oxygen Cost of Aerobic Bench Stepping at Three Heights," *Journal of Strength & Conditioning Research,* 7, 163-167.
16. Calcarco et al.
17. K. Greenlaw, et al., "The Energy cost of Traditional Versus Power Bench Step Exercise at Heights of Four, Six, and Eight Inches," *Medicine and Science in Sport and Exercise,* 27, 5 (June 1995, supplement), abstrace #1343.
18. M. Scharff-Olsen, et al., "Physiological Responses of Males and Females to Bench Step at Two Different Rates," *Sports Medicine,* 3 (1996): 164-175.
19. Scharff-Olsen.
20. Len, M. A. Kravitz, and Rich Deivert, "The Safe Way to Step," *IDEA Today,* April, 1991, pp. 47-50.
21. Lorna Francis, et al., p. 20.
22. M. Groupe-Kennedy, "Managing Step Intensity," *ACE Certified News,* 2:5 (1997), p. 9.
23. Lorna Francis et al., p. 20.
24. Step Reebok Guidelines, ACE Chapter 9, p. 277
25. Len Kravitz, et al., p. 48.
26. Douglas H. Richie, Jr., "How to Choose Shoes," *IDEA Today,* April 1991, p. 67.
27. Richie.
28. American College of Obsetricians & Gynocologists, *Safety Guidelines for Women Who Exercise* (ACOG Home Exercise Programs no. 2). (Washington DC: ACOG, 1986), p. 6.
29. ACOG, pp. 4- 5.

### ▆▆ Chapter 4

1. Candice Copeland-Brooks *Moves . . . and More!* [videotape] (San Diego: IDEA, Inc., 1990).
2. Candice Copeland *The Low-Impact Challenger For The Fitness Professional* [videotape] (Newark, NJ: PPI Entertainment Group/ Parade Video, 1991).
3. Julie Moo-Bradley & Jerrie Moo-Thurman *Aerobics Choreography in Action: The High-Low Impact Advantage* [videotape] (San Diego: IDEA, Inc., 1990).
4. Lynne Brick *Total Body Workout* [videotape] (Philadelphia: Creative Instructors Aerobics, 1991).
5. Amy Jones, "Point-Counterpoint. Sequencing a Dance-Exercise Class," *Dance Exercise Today,* May/June 1985.
6. Lorna Francis, Peter Francis, and Gin Miller, *Step-Reebok, The First Aerobic Training Workout With Muscle: Instructor Training Manual.* (Reebok International, 1990), p. 23.

7. Len Kravitz, et al., "Static & PNF Stretches," *IDEA Today,* March 1990.
8. Kravitz.
9. Kravitz.
10. Kravitz.

### ▆▆ Chapter 5

1. Karen Mazzeo, *Aerobics: The Way To Fitness* (Englewood, CO: 1992), pp. 95–104.
2. Lorna Francis, Peter Francis, and Gin Miller, *Step-Reebok, The First Aerobic Training Workout With Muscle: Instructor Training Manual* (Reebok International Ltd., 1990), p. 25.
3. Francis et al., p. 25.
4. Candice Copeland-Brooks, *Moves . . . and More!* [videotape] (San Diego: IDEA, Inc. 1990).

### ▆▆ Chapter 6

1. Candice Copeland-Brooks, "Smooth Moves," *IDEA Today.* June 1991, p. 34.
2. Lorna Francis, Peter Francis, and Gin Miller, *Step-Reebok, The First Aerobic Training Workout With Muscle: Instructor Training Manual.* Reebok International Ltd., 1990), p. 26.
3. Copeland-Brooks, p. 34.
4. Copeland-Brooks.
5. Tamilee Webb, M.A., "Step 'Q' Signs," *IDEA Fitness Renaissance Educational Conference and Fitness Expo* (Pittsburg, PA: 1991).
6. Lynn Brick, R.N., "Step I.T.," *IDEA Fitness Renaissance Educational Conference and Fitness Expo* (Pittsburg, PA: 1991).
7. Lorna Francis, Peter Francis, and Gin Miller, *Step-Reebok, The First Aerobic Training Workout With Muscle: Instructor Training Manual.* Reebok International Ltd., 1990.
8. Joan Price, "Stepping Basics," *IDEA Today,* November/December, 1990, p. 57.
9. Ralph La Forge, "What the Latest Research Has to Say About Step Exercise," *IDEA Today,* September, 1991, p. 33,
10. L. Calarco, et al., "The Metabolic Cost of Six Common Movement Patterns of Bench Step Aerobic Dance," *Medicine and Science in Sports and Exercise* (abstract), 23: 4 (April 1991), S140.
11. Gin Miller, "Taking the Right Step," *IDEA Today,* October, 1991, pp. 36-39.
12. Diane Chapman, "Two-Stepping Takes Off," *IDEA Today* (Industry News), September 1992, p. 11.

### ▆▆ Chapter 7

1. L. Giteck, "Circuit Training," *Fitness Management,* August 1997, pp. 31–34.
2. T. DeMond, "Reach New Limits with Interval Training," *IDEA Today,* April 1992, pp. 27–29.
3. L. Kravitz, et al., "The Physiological Benefits of a Combined Step & Aerobics Training Program," edited by J. Rippe, *IDEA World Research Forum,* Las Vegas, 1992.

4. A. Perry, et al., "A Physiological Comparison of Interval vs. Continuous Aerobic Dance Training," *Medicine and Science in Sports & Exercise,* 19: 2 (April 1987).

5. "Interval Training," *ACE FitnessMatters,* 3: 6. (Nov./Dec. 1997), 2.

6. Reebok University *Slide Reebok Manual,* Reebok Alliance 1-800-325-7692.

7. *Slide News,* Fall 1993, Fitness Innovations Inc. , 9 Russell Rd., Winchester, MA 01890.

8. Reebok University.

9. K. Hargarten, "A Rope-Jumping Class," *IDEA Today,* March 1989.

10. B. Bellinger, et al. "Energy Expenditure of a Non Contact Boxing Training Session Compared with Submaximal Treadmill Running," *Medicine & Science in Sport & Exercise,* 29: 12 (1997), 1653–1656.

11. E. Rodriguiez, "Putting the Punch in Your Boxing Classes," *IDEA Health & Fitness Source,* June 1998, pp. 23–28.

12. Lorna Francis, "Moderate-Impact Aerobics," also, *Aerobics Choreography* (San Diego: IDEA, Association for Fitness Professionals, 1990).

### Chapter 8

1. *In Step*, Reebok Newsletter, Spring 1992, p. 10.

2. Greg Niederlander, *Step Strength* [videotape]. (SPRI Products & Brick Bodies 1991).

3. American College of Sports Medicine's *Resource Manual, Guidelines for Exercise Testing and Prescription,* 3d edition, (Baltimore: Williams and Wilkins, 1998).

4. *The Step, Introduction to Step Training* [videotape] (Atlanta: Sports Step, Inc., 1989).

5. James L. Hesson, *Weight Training For Life* (Englewood, CO: Morton Publishing, 1985), Appendices pp. 164–165.

6. Karen S. Mazzeo, *Aerobics: The Way To Fitness* (Englewood, CO: Morton Publishing, 1992), p. 51.

7. *Pumping Rubber,* SPRI Products, Inc., 507 N. Wolf Road, Wheeling, IL 60090. (instructions for product use, 1988; 1-800-222-7774).

8. *Pumping Rubber.*

9. *Pumping Rubber.*

10. American College of Obstetricians and Gynecologists, *Safety Guidelines for Women Who Exercise* (ACOG Home Exercise Programs) (Washington, DC: ACOG, 1986), p.6.

11. Hesson, p. 33.

12. Hesson.

13. Lynn Brick, "Step I.T.," IDEA Fitness Renaissance Educational Conference and Fitness Expo, Pittsburg, 1991.

14. John Patrick O'Shea, *Scientific Principles and Methods of Strength Fitness,* 2d edition (Reading, MA: Addison-Wesley, 1976), p. 89.

### Chapter 9

1. Bernie Rabin, educational and clinical psychologist, yearly guest speaker to Karen S. Mazzeo's Tension Management and Health Methods courses, Bowling Green State University, 1978–1988.

2. Shad Helmstetter, *What To Say When You Talk To Yourself* (New York: Pocket Books/Simon & Schuster, 1986), p. 98.

3. Karen S. Mazzeo, *Stress\*Time\*Life Management Principles, Methods, and Assessment Techniques* (Bowling Green, OH: Mazzeo Reprographics, 1998) p. 42.

### Chapter 10

1. Nutrition Education Services, *Pyramid Plus, A Star-Studded Guide to Food Choices for Better Health* (Portland: Oregon Dairy Council, 1997).

2. Judy Tillapaugh, "Cross-Training in the Kitchen," *IDEA Today,* October 1991, p. 21.

3. U. S. Department of Agriculture, *Food Guide Pyramid, A Guide to Daily Food Choices* (Washington, DC: Government Printing Office 1992).

4. Nutrition Education Services.

5. American Dietetics Association, http://.www.eatright.org/adap1197.html #2, Hot Topics section, Position Papers, "Position of the American Dietetics Association: Vegetarian Diets," pp. 12–13.

6. American Institute for Cancer Research Newsletter, "Water Down Your Summer Thirst", 60 (Summer 1998), 5.

7. Gatorade Company (division of Quaker Oats Company) "Fluid Pyramid" pamphlet (1-800-884-2867).

8. Nutrition Education Services.

9. Nutrition Education Services.

10. National Dairy Council, *"Guide to Wise Food Choices"* (B 170-1) (Rosemont, IL: National Dairy Council, 1978), p.1.

11. Nutrition Education Services.

12. Nutrition Education Services.

13. U. S. Department of Agriculture, Human Nutrition Information Service, *Home & Garden Bulletin,* No. 253-2, p.5, July 1993 (Washington, DC: Government Printing Office).

14. USDA, *Home & Garden Bulletin,* Numbers 253–1 through 253–8.

15. American Dietetics Association, http://www.eatright.org/adap 1197.html#2, pp. 1–18.

16. Tammy Kime-Sheets, author of original teaching tool entitled, "How To Eat Without The Meat", in the section 'Cut The Animal Fat', p. 2, distributed to clients at Nutrition Wellness seminars and workshops in the greater Toledo, Ohio area, 1998.

17. Tammy Kime-Sheets, p. 2.

18. Vegetarian Resource Group, http://vrg.org/nutrition/ ada-paper.htm, pp.1–3.

19. Tammy Kime-Sheets, p. 2.

20. Vegetarian Resource Group, pp. 1–3.

21. American Dietetics Association, pp. 11–12.

22. American Dietetics Association, pp. 6–7.

23. American Institute for Cancer Research Newsletter, p. 5.

24. American Institute for Cancer Research Newsletter, p. 5.

25. Tammy Kime-Sheets, *W.I.C. Wellness News...You Can Use!* "W.A.T.E.R. = Water A 'Treat' Everyone Requires"; "Water-The Perfect Drink!"; "Water Replacement Plan" (W.I.C. Fulton/Henry County, OH), August 1997.

26. American Institute for Cancer, Research Newsletter, p. 5.

27. Jan Lewis, "Nutrition Notes: Nutrition and the Athlete," Workshop Series, Nutrition Education and Training Program, Bowling Green State University, Bowling Green, OH, 1981.

28. Mayo Clinic Diet and Nutrition Resource Center, http://www.mayo.ivi.com/mayo/common/htm/diet page.htm, Mayo Health O@sis section, "Energy gels—At the competitive edge," p. 2.

29. Mayo Clinic Diet and Nutrition Resource Center, p. 2.

30. USDA, *Home & Garden Bulletin,* Numbers 253–1 through 253–258.

31. Lucy M. Williams, lecture and literature, "Shopping Tips for Low-Fat, Low-Salt, Low Cholesterol Diets," delivered to Karen S. Mazzeo's Anchor Fitness-Personal Excellence class, February, 1991.

32. Williams.

33. USDA, *Home & Garden Bulletin,* Number 253–8, p. 2.

### ▬▬ Chapter 11

1. Werner W. K.Hoeger, *Principles & Labs for Physical Fitness & Wellness* (Englewood, CO: Morton Publishing, 1994), pp. 49–64.

2. Tufts University Nutrition Navigator http://navigator.tufts.edu/profess.html, About The Ratings section, pp. 1–2, and Health Professionals section.

3 Linda Stonecipher, *Issues In Contemporary Nutrition, Current and Controversial Readings with Links to Relevant Web Sites,* (Englewood, CO: Morton Publishing, 1998) pp. 201–210.

4. Jan Lewis, *Nutrition Notes. Dietary Guidelines 2,* Bowling Green State University, Bowling Green, OH, 1981.

5. Dr. Steven Blair, keynote speaker at American Alliance for Health, Physical Education, Recreation, & Dance National Convention, Indianapolis, 1992.

6. Connirae Andreas and Steven A. Andreas, *Heart of the Mind* (Moab, UT: Real People Press, 1989), p. 251.

7. Connirae Andreas, p. 125.

8. Jan Lewis, p. 6.

9. Jan Lewis, p. 4.

10. Lewis.

11. Lewis.

# INDEX

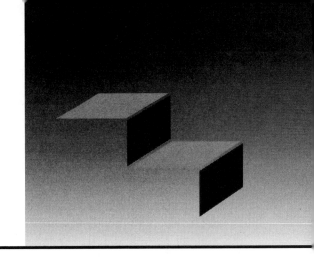